Penguin B

REVIVE

Jill Thomas is a naturopath, herbalist and iridologist and runs Albert Park Naturopathic Centre, a busy practice in inner Melbourne. She has lectured at the Melbourne College of Natural Medicine (MCNM) for the past five years and has spent a year as the resident naturopath at a Melbourne radio station. She has won numerous awards for clinical excellence in nutrition and herbal medicine, and graduated as dux of her year at the MCNM. Jill insists that despite a busy schedule she remains un-exhausted due to daily therapeutic doses of B vitamins, various herbal tonics and regular excursions to the cinema to see a good French film.

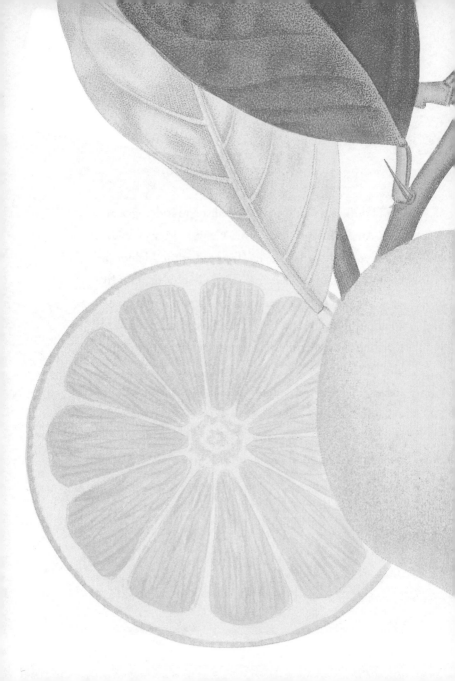

Revive

HOW TO OVERCOME
FATIGUE NATURALLY

⁓

Jill Thomas N.D.

Penguin Books

PENGUIN BOOKS

Published by the Penguin Group
Penguin Group (Australia)
250 Camberwell Road, Camberwell, Victoria 3124, Australia
(a division of Pearson Australia Group Pty Ltd)
Penguin Group (USA) Inc.
375 Hudson Street, New York, New York 10014, USA
Penguin Group (Canada)
90 Eglinton Avenue East, Suite 700, Toronto, ON M4P 2Y3, Canada
(a division of Pearson Penguin Canada Inc.)
Penguin Books Ltd
80 Strand, London WC2R 0RL, England
Penguin Ireland
25 St Stephen's Green, Dublin 2, Ireland
(a division of Penguin Books Ltd)
Penguin Books India Pvt Ltd
11 Community Centre, Panchsheel Park, New Delhi – 110 017, India
Penguin Group (NZ)
Cnr Airborne and Rosedale Roads, Albany, Auckland, New Zealand
(a division of Pearson New Zealand Ltd)
Penguin Books (South Africa) (Pty) Ltd
24 Sturdee Avenue, Rosebank, Johannesburg 2196, South Africa

Penguin Books Ltd, Registered Offices: 80 Strand, London, WC2R 0RL, England

First published by Penguin Group (Australia), a division of Pearson Australia Group Pty Ltd, 2005

10 9 8 7 6 5 4 3 2 1

Cover and text design by Elizabeth Dias © Penguin Group (Australia)
Cover illustration 'Limonier Mellarose' lemon (*Citrus limonia*) by Antoine Risso/Porteau, RHS Lindley Library
Author photograph by Jodie Hutchinson
Typeset in 12.25/16.75 pt Adobe Garamond by Post Pre-press Group, Brisbane, Queensland
Printed in Australia by McPherson's Printing Group, Maryborough, Victoria

National Library of Australia
Cataloguing-in-Publication data:

Thomas, Jill.
  Revive.

  Bibliography.
  Includes index.
  ISBN 0 14 300336 4.

  1. Fatigue. 2. Fatigue – Prevention. 3. Self-care, Health. I. Title.

616.047

www.penguin.com.au

For Janine, A Very Nice Type
REVIVE would not have been possible without you!

The case histories I refer to throughout the book are those of actual clients I have seen over the years; however, their names and personal circumstances have been changed to protect their privacy and for reasons of client confidentiality.

Thank you to Martin & Pleasance for graciously granting permission to reproduce their Bach flowers guide.

Every attempt has been made to acknowledge source material. The author and publisher would be pleased to hear from any source whose work has not been acknowledged.

ACKNOWLEDGEMENTS

With thanks and gratitude to Thresherman's Bakery, especially Maria and Sam, for providing a sunny spot, a friendly environment and sound nourishment to help me maintain the writing momentum.

A big, warm thank you to all the team at St Vincent Place Medical Centre. Your friendship and support have always been invaluable . . . I promise, no more moaning about publishers' deadlines.

CONTENTS

CHAPTER ONE

WELCOME TO REVIVE

Bounce out of bed each morning with a positive spring in your step; greet the day with enthusiasm and happiness; move into the mid-afternoon with a clear head and sufficient energy to sustain you adequately until the end of your working day; and complete each day feeling pleasantly tired and relaxed enough to enjoy a deep, peaceful, uninterrupted and rejuvenating sleep. This is within the reach of us all and, indeed, is the normal human condition.

Health is not a concrete state we attain once and for all. We don't get there and remain there, as if curled up complacently in a comfortable chair, never having to make an effort to get up again and go about our daily tasks. Our ability to decide to move out of that chair towards even better health and even greater energy is a fortunate human capacity indeed. It means we are able to direct our health, to change our circumstances and improve our situation. Health is a fluid, dynamic condition and, in the main, *we* are in charge.

This is an exciting concept: we have the freedom to choose to turn our state of health around. Given the right information, a little direction and with a certain enthusiastic commitment, *we* can undo that tiredness and decide to create a life sparkling with energy once again.

Tick box for vitality

- Do you wake up refreshed each morning?
- Do you feel mentally alert, have precision in thought and action and a strong memory?
- Do you rarely come down with colds and flus?
- Do you start and end each day energetically and enthusiastically?
- Do you have sufficient energy to complete all your daily tasks?
- Are you just as mentally precise at three o'clock in the afternoon as you are at nine o'clock in the morning?
- Do you have a strong appetite and feel hungry at meal times?
- Do you fall asleep within thirty minutes and sleep soundly?

If you answered no to any of these questions then REVIVE can provide you with some easy answers. Together we shall examine ways to beat fatigue permanently by using safe, simple, natural methods.

You will discover in the following chapters a friendly discussion of the positive role that diet, nutrition, herbal medicine and lifestyle – such as exercise, meditation and sleep management – have in creating and maintaining abundant energy. This is the natural state of being and, unless we are suffering from some very serious health concerns, we can and should expect to live every day of our lives in a state of positive energy. So, let's not waste time *not* experiencing vitality, all of the time.

Throughout the years I have been in practice, nothing has been more inspiring and genuinely satisfying than seeing a tired, listless and mildly anxious patient transform into an energetic individual positively glowing with vitality and good health. And it is really quite easy to achieve.

A valuable way to approach this book is to read through all the chapters and then return to those areas that are especially relevant to you. If, for example, you conclude that your fatigue is mainly a result of unwise dietary choices, poor sleeping patterns and, perhaps, escalating food allergies, then return to those sections and make notes of the measures you need to specifically apply to your daily routine in order to put an end once and for all to your tiredness.

In CHAPTER FIFTEEN you will find an easy-to-follow summary of my anti-fatigue regime. I urge you to photocopy this, adding any personal measures *you* may need to take. Stick these guidelines to your fridge door or place them in your diary and apply these measures with great commitment for a minimum of six weeks and preferably up to three months. If you have been diligent in your approach (no cheating!), I can guarantee there will be a discernable, highly motivating and energising improvement.

We truly can become what we aspire to, so let's enthusiastically embrace the goal of overcoming fatigue permanently and see where it takes us. A much more comfortable spot for sure, where energy is in abundance *not* in short supply.

Let's commit to vitality!

CHAPTER TWO

IDENTIFYING FATIGUE

In a sad, quiet voice at the end of a consultation I often hear, 'And by the way, Jill, I'm always tired.' I have heard this unhappy statement a thousand times. If we dig carefully beneath most people's general health concerns, we find a deep, underlying tiredness. A national fatigue. A widespread, international exhaustion. This begs the question, why? And, more importantly, it requires an answer. What safe, simple, effective means can we use to overcome fatigue permanently?

Fatigue is not a disorder. It is often mistaken for one, but it is, in fact, a *symptom*. It may be the earliest symptom of a number of health problems such as anaemia, a sluggish thyroid gland, systemic candida infection, adrenal gland exhaustion, hypoglycaemia or viral infection, such as glandular fever. Contributing factors often include lack of exercise, depression, dehydration, insomnia, a vitamin

B complex or magnesium deficiency caused by dietary inadequacies, or multiple food allergies. Unrelenting and disabling fatigue is the main symptom of chronic fatigue syndrome (CFS).

Persistent or even intermittent tiredness that is not caused by any underlying illness, however, is often simply the result of poor choices – an unhealthy diet and unwise lifestyle habits. The combination of a diet overly abundant in refined carbohydrates and stimulants, such as caffeine, alcohol and nicotine, mixed together with a fair dollop of emotional stress, is a recipe for part-time and possibly full-time exhaustion. However, since tiredness can so frequently be attributed to wrong choices, we have complete control over our recovery. This is a liberating thought indeed.

British physician Thomas McKeown wrote, 'It is assumed that we are ill and made well, but it is nearer the truth to say we are well and are made ill.' He is right, you know, and if we can make ourselves unwell, we can certainly make ourselves well again. We simply need to make better-informed and sensible decisions about everything that enters our mouth and the way we choose to live our lives.

Vitality is our natural state of being. Devitalisation, or fatigue, is the antithesis of good health. The more run down we are and the greater our stress, the less well we feel and the further devitalised we become; and sadly many people decide to stay there. Returning to a state of equilibrium may take only a matter of weeks to a couple of months to achieve; or for the seriously run down it may be a matter of many months. However, constant attention to promoting one's health nearly always results in a new vital being. Never give up – there is always an answer to overcoming fatigue.

Realistically, we do not exist in an ideal world where moderation always rules. There are often periods in our lives when due to work, family or study commitments we work exceedingly long hours and lose valuable sleep; consequently, we feel the full effects of stress and anxiety. Paradoxically, it is often at these times of *increased* nutritional needs that our diet becomes less than ideal and we do not exercise sufficiently. Indeed, the cumulative effect of multiple stressors can combine to create a total stress load that has serious physical and emotional implications.

However, whatever the cause of fatigue – anaemia, Epstein-Barr virus, hypoglycaemia, post-viral syndrome (the 'never been well since' syndrome), or a vitamin B deficiency – these are all manifestations of a severely depleted 'vital capacity', and profound fatigue has an overwhelming requirement for restorative measures.

SIGNS AND SYMPTOMS OF FATIGUE

In clinical practice there are a number of criteria that can be drawn on to assess the general state of the body's energy reserves.

A person is said to have depleted vital capacity if more than one of the following symptoms apply:

* undue and prolonged fatigue, listlessness and possible muscle weakness; especially if combined with tension and irritability
* a tendency for sleep to be broken in the early hours of the morning
* waking up tired and unrefreshed
* night sweating
* chronically raised lymph glands
* weak digestive function and poor assimilation; vague, persistent nausea and abdominal discomfort; low appetite or escalating food intolerances
* an awareness of being continuously below par; of not being able to fire on all cylinders, despite a desire to do so.

Recapturing your old self, or substituting a new energetic one, is not hard. Changes in diet, lifestyle and attitude are often all that is required, and that is easy. It is frequently just a matter of making a decision and a commitment to change, plus perhaps some gentle professional guidance along the way to direct you onto the right road.

A female patient, Meredith, aged thirty-eight, sought treatment for an uncharacteristic lack of stamina, general malaise and poor sleep. Her bowels had also become sluggish over the past twelve months, with a tendency to slight constipation and incomplete bowel movements. She worked as a team leader with a national banking organisation, had a busy social life and was reasonably physically active. She was able to manage on the whole, but found that one too many late nights, or increased demands and deadlines at work, would result in several days of complete and utter exhaustion when all she could do was come home, eat dinner and crawl into bed by 8.30 p.m. She would then have a restless night's sleep, waking unrefreshed and tired the next morning. This had become a pattern for the past sixteen months.

Meredith presented as quite pale with dark circles beneath her eyes and the sclera, or whites of her eyes, was red and bloodshot (often a sign of food allergies). Her voice had, unsurprisingly, a tired resigned tone. Her iris analysis revealed mild adrenal exhaustion, physiological stress and an under-active digestive system. She frequently skipped breakfast or else grabbed a muesli bar on the way to work, lunch was a ham and cheese sandwich (double proteins, but more of that later) and dinner was more often than not take-away or else cheese on toast. She drank three to four coffees a day and four glasses of water. Meredith's water consumption was not unusual. 'Not enough' is the response I commonly receive to my standard naturopathic question of 'How much water do you drink each day?'

Meredith was placed on a herbal regime, a good-quality mega-dose vitamin B complex, plus a magnesium supplement. She was asked to increase her water consumption to 1½ litres daily, to eat an oat-based breakfast and to incorporate more fresh fruits and vegetables into her diet. A brisk walk of 45–50 minutes each day was also suggested. The first few weeks saw a mild improvement in symptoms: the mid-afternoon slump disappeared and sleep improved at night. By the eighth week she felt the herbs were definitely helping, digestion had improved and she was now waking refreshed and feeling like her old self. After twelve weeks the herbs were decreased and eventually phased out, and Meredith's improved diet took over as the basis to her sustained recovery.

So, what can we do to make sure we have adequate resources at times of increased need, and, at the same time, obtain maximum benefits from our diet when our lives are generally running smoothly? That is, how can we both prevent and address sub-optimal health? What habits can we build into our lives to ensure that vitality is a normal part of our everyday experience?

Let's begin by examining four essential components that we can adapt to our individual requirements, to help both *prevent* and *alleviate* chronic tiredness and persistent fatigue.

DIET

Health is found at the end of a knife and fork. The importance of a nutritionally dense diet cannot be emphasised enough. Everything is made from something. Carbohydrates, proteins and essential fatty acids (EFAs) provide the vitamins, minerals, enzymes and amino acids our bodies require to be fully functional. Muscles, bones, tissues, hormones, hair, skin, nails and organs, including the brain, are all made from and totally dependent on the nutrients derived from our diet. The way we move, think, respond and look is a reflection of what we choose to place in our mouth. Food for thought indeed! Even the hormones produced by stress, as well as the tissues that make them, require adequate nutrition. It is impossible to be truly healthy without a nutritionally sound diet.

VITAMINS AND MINERALS

All the B-group vitamins, especially vitamins B5 (pantothenic acid) and B6 (pyridoxine), plus vitamin C and the minerals calcium, magnesium and potassium, are extremely important in addressing stress, which is a key factor in fatigue. The very same nutrients, with the addition of iron and, especially, coenzyme Q10 (CoQ10), are equally important in alleviating chronic tiredness. They are all key components involved in the production of energy at a cellular level. We can also use particular vitamins and amino acids to increase mental alertness and combat brain fatigue.

HERBS

There are many herbs that play an important role in fatigue management, and we are fortunate to have a magnificent selection in the herbal kingdom to choose from. Some herbs, such as oats, vervain and skullcap, are soothing and restorative in nature, and specifically address stress and anxiety.

Another group of herbs, the 'adaptogens', enable us to adapt effectively to physiological changes caused by stress. Herbs such as Siberian ginseng, withania and gota kola are extremely important in the management and treatment of fatigue. Siberian ginseng, for example, contains plant glycosides (sugars) that act on the adrenal glands to help prevent adrenal hypertrophy (enlargement) and excessive adrenal hormone production. It also increases energy and stamina and helps the body resist viral infections. Other herbs, such as bacopa and ginkgo, improve our mental agility and memory recall.

LIFESTYLE
Exercise

The nutritional components of a healthy diet are only as good as the blood supply that carries them to our tissues, and an effective way to optimise circulation is exercise. Exercise also means enhanced transfer of oxygen to the cells, and we all know how even a minor oxygen deficit can affect our brain cells and contribute enormously to fatigue. The range of active possibilities is endless; there's always an enjoyable solution to overcome our inner exercise saboteur. Moreover, the proven beneficial effect of exercise on mood and depression (let alone its toning effect on muscle tissue!) is further encouragement to lace up those runners and get moving. Exercise can be imaginatively combined with various interesting meditation techniques to produce some very happy results.

Insomnia

Night after night of poor-quality sleep does not promote days full of enthusiasm or abundant energy, and it certainly does not encourage bouncing out of bed for an early morning work-out. A chronic sleep deficit can result in overwhelming fatigue.

Even one night of poor sleep results in a less than productive day, but an accumulation of restless nights can snowball into foggy days and, if it becomes chronic, fatigued months. If sleep has become a health issue there are many, many measures that can be taken to break the sleep-deprivation cycle and help return us to sound restorative sleep. Herbal medicine is particularly useful in re-establishing sleep patterns; the B-group vitamins, together with minerals such as calcium and magnesium, plus amino acids such as tryptophan all have a role to play here.

Focused attention

Meditation helps quieten the mind by stopping the incessant mental chatter that so often prevents us from falling asleep or wakes us in the early hours. It also soothes and calms an irritated nervous system and provides the ideal environment in which a healthy diet, sound nutrition and herbal medicine can work their restorative wonders. A restless, busy mind that never stops darting here and there, always thinking ahead, rarely giving us a quiet moment, is exhausting. Herbs and the Bach flower remedies can be used, if necessary, to help establish a calmer state to get our meditation off the ground – so to speak! A quiet mind is an excellent base from which to leap back into glowing vitality.

So, what can we do to overcome fatigue and ensure optimal vitality? Let's start with diet.

CHAPTER THREE

Diet — a revival plan

Obtaining optimal nourishment

To paraphrase Henry Thoreau, 'Your body is your temple, treat it wisely'. This is very sound advice. Everything we put into our mouths becomes part of us. Every cell in our body is made from and energised by the nutritional substances derived from the foods we eat. This is a profound concept.

Fundamentally, we can view ourselves as one large cell, or as a coherent mass of cells, with all the functions of a cell enlarged. We are as healthy as each of our individual cells, and we have 60 billion of them to maintain in good functioning order. We do this by the food we eat, and that is a challenging thought! These cells must be well nourished if we are going to look and feel vibrant. Skin, hair, eyes, lips, nails – our outward self – mirror the tissues from which they grow and are composed.

I am sure we have all experienced the frightening sight of our face in the mirror the morning after a night of overindulgence, or following a day of overconsumption of the foods we know we are sensitive to. A regular client of mine is guaranteed to wake up with a bloated face, multiple creases beneath her eyes and puffy upper eyelids if she eats too many yeast-containing foods. An example of this would be toast and Vegemite for breakfast; focaccia for lunch; and for dinner, pasta with a rich tomato and mushroom sauce accompanied by a crusty French baguette, or a takeaway pizza or Turkish bread. On a more positive note, we also know how fantastic we look and feel after following a gentle elimination diet or a liver-friendly regime for a week or two: clear, sparkling eyes, shiny hair, radiant skin and, to top it off, mental clarity as well.

FOOD AS ENERGY

What is food? A simple answer is that food is fuel, consumed to produce energy. Most of this energy is used to maintain a complex array of essential bodily functions, such as breathing, digestion and elimination. Excess energy derived from food, as a result of overconsumption and under-expenditure, is stored away as fat.

Nutrition can never be unimportant. Food and its constituents – vitamins, minerals and amino acids – provide energy and undertake this vital work at the cellular level. Some foods, such as wheatgerm, yeast, oats, leafy green vegetables and blackstrap molasses, due to their nutritional profile also contain an 'anti-stress factor'.

The biggest dietary mistake we can make when fatigued is to consume too many refined carbohydrates, and stimulants such as coffee, tea, alcohol and caffeine-containing soft drinks. Not only does this type of diet contribute to fatigue but it also contains very little in the way of nutrition. Too much sugar sends blood-sugar levels skyrocketing and then plummeting, often resulting in reactive hypoglycaemia (consequential low blood-sugar levels) and a guaranteed energy slump or, more seriously, a shaky crash in the mid-afternoon. Hypoglycaemia can be controlled by the mineral chromium, often combined with other minerals and vitamins in a formula known as Glucose Tolerance Factors, but ideally it shouldn't come to that. Blood-sugar levels should, in the first place, be controlled by diet. The glycaemic index (GI), which many of you will have heard of, is an indicator of the effect that carbohydrates have, after ingestion, on sugar levels in the blood. We should aim to choose foods that have only a moderate or reduced insulin response (see APPENDIX ONE Glycaemic index).

Stimulants, such as caffeine and alcohol, rob us of

key nutrients via their diuretic action, as well as increasing our need for nutrients involved in the production of key neurotransmitters. Neurotransmitters are chemicals that carry information from one nerve cell to another, enabling the brain to receive and send messages. Some neurotransmitters you may be familiar with are: endorphins, enkephalin, melatonin, dopamine and serotonin. All together, about fifty substances are either known or strongly suspected to be neurotransmitters. The secondary impact of stimulants on our wellbeing is via their effect on the liver and hence the detoxification process. A liver which is severely compromised is unable to adequately break down undesirable substances and thereby increases the body's total toxic load. This is tiring.

USING WATER WISELY

Drinking the right amount of water is vital to good health. Water is absolutely essential to the life in our cells as almost every bodily process needs water. Water dissolves and transports the nutrients required for metabolism. It takes water to chew and digest food, to create blood, to move muscles, to breathe, to think – we would have to agree these are fairly essential functions! Two-thirds of our body's weight is water, and we lose approximately 2 litres a day: through the skin (25 per cent), urine (50 per cent), lungs (20 per cent) and faeces (5 per cent).

A scientific formula for calculating precisely how much water we require is: 35 ml of water per kilo of body weight. Therefore, someone who weighs 50 kg needs to drink approximately 1.75 litres of water per day. (A little more than is commonly considered adequate!) Of course, the amount of water we require is also influenced by our activity level, the climate and our diet.

A recent response I received from a client on asking him how much water he drank each day was, 'Oh, I drink about two glasses of water per day, but I also drink about 1½ litres of fruit juice and 1½ litres of tea each day.' Oh dear! There is a common misunderstanding about the difference in benefits between various fluids. Tea and coffee are dehydrating, and the sugar in this amount of fruit juice is clearly too much. We should eat our fruits, not drink them, and for every cup of tea or coffee add two glasses of water.

On the other hand, I remember counselling a client on her excessive water consumption (now, this is unusual); she was drinking 6 litres of water a day and weighed approximately 49 kg. The toll on her kidneys was dangerous and the systemic effects potentially lethal (brain swelling, confusion, seizures, coma).

Water is ideally consumed at several intervals

throughout the day: one or two glasses on waking up and then about an hour before each meal. Water should not be drunk with meals as it dilutes digestive enzymes and therefore affects digestion and nutrient assimilation. It should be drunk at room temperature, never icy cold from the refrigerator because this stuns digestive enzymes. In winter, when most of us experience difficulty drinking the required daily amount, try sipping glasses of warm water with a slice of lemon or lime.

A CHEMISTRY LESSON IN CHEWING . . . GOODBYE TO THE GULP!

The breakdown of carbohydrates begins in the mouth. The salivary enzyme amylase (ptyalin) starts the very important process of breaking down starches as they begin their journey to the small intestine for absorption. It may astonish you to learn that the three pairs of salivary glands found in our mouth together secrete about a litre of water a day. Let's not waste this water. After all, using water wisely should be entrenched in our psyche by now! The water in saliva provides a medium for dissolving foods so they can be tasted and therefore initiate other digestive reactions. The salivary amylase in the swallowed food continues to act on starches for another 15–30 minutes in the stomach.

Chewing our food properly is just as important as the type of food we decide to place in our mouths. Gulping our meals will result in poor absorption of the nutrients we need to produce energy, as well as abdominal distention, pain and bloating. Impairment of nutrient absorption, due to insufficient chewing, means that proteins, fats, minerals and vitamins are absorbed more slowly and in smaller amounts.

Another enzyme found in saliva is lingual lipase, which is secreted by glands beneath the tongue. This enzyme, which is active in the stomach, digests as much as 30 per cent of dietary triglycerides into fatty acids.

Chewing well not only breaks up our food into small, easy-to-handle particles, it also ensures that saliva and enzymes are mixed well with the food, and protects the mucosa of the pharynx and oesophagus as it makes its way down to the stomach. Thirty chews per mouthful is a good place to begin. Concentrate on everything you put into your mouth: taste it, chew it, savour it and *relax* at the same time.

Eating in a calm, relaxed manner automatically slows down our individual eating style and enhances digestion. Recently I watched in horror from the bench of my favourite inner-city cafe as a young man literally shoved spoonfuls of meat and pasta into his mouth at a startlingly rapid rate.

He certainly didn't seem to be enjoying his food, it was simply fuel. Within five minutes a very large plate of a heavy lunchtime meal had been shovelled in, completely by-passing his salivary enzymes. I can guarantee this young man would have returned to work with a belly ache, feeling bloated and tired, having absorbed precious little nutritional value from his gigantic meal. He polished off his lunch with a can of Coke, completing the gaseous abdominal mess well. I was tempted to leap from my window seat and give him a few helpful eating tips; however, this was a man with a mission and I felt that naturopathic interference would not be warmly welcomed. I even had some digestive enzymes in my handbag (as every good naturopath would), which certainly would have provided some immediate relief.

Even our vocabulary and choice of words reflect our busy 21st-century-attitude towards meals and eating behaviour. How often do we hear ourselves saying, 'I'm going to grab a bite to eat.'? Grabbing lunch hardly evokes visions of eating peacefully. Even worse are the advertised 'quick meals', guaranteed to get you in and out of a restaurant in record time. This is a frightening trend.

Yes, food is fuel, but as human beings we have the luxury of making food a lifestyle choice. The celebration of eating is a very human trait: relaxing with friends over a meal of good food and conversation, or sitting alone, with a candle burning, giving thanks and thought to the food we are slowly eating and enjoying is a civilised and sensible approach to meals. A far cry from the shovel technique. Thank goodness for the emerging 'slow food' trend and the consequential expansion of the flavour palate!

ACID VS ALKALINE

Our diet should ideally be 70 per cent alkaline and 30 per cent acidic. The pH of our blood plasma needs to remain at a pretty constant 7.41. Even a slight deviation either way can have deadly serious consequences for our health – for example an acid pH of 6.95 results in diabetic coma.

The acid/alkaline balance of our blood depends largely on what we consume: foods are either acid-forming or alkaline-forming. Generally, those that leave an alkaline residue are the fresh fruits, and green and yellow vegetables. Foods that increase acidity are almost all the rest: meat; cheese; eggs; nuts (except almonds); legumes; seeds; grain foods, such as bread, pasta, rice and cereals; refined sugar; coffee and tea. Millet, buckwheat and soy beans (tofu) are an exception, being alkaline-producing grains and legumes. Yoghurt is also alkaline.

One of the biggest mistakes in nutrition is the assumption that acidic fruits, like citrus, pineapples and tomatoes, are acid-forming. In fact, during metabolism their organic acids are broken down to release energy and the acidic end-product, carbon dioxide, is breathed out leaving a residue of alkaline minerals.

It is far easier to become over-acidic than it is to become over-alkaline. The standard Western diet is, unfortunately, rather acidic – think refined foods, fats, animal proteins and sugar. Anxiety, worry and lack of sleep also result in an acidic constitution; as does the consumption of many 'standard' pharmaceutical drugs.

A sour taste in the mouth in the morning can be the first sign that we are entering an acidic-overload. A diet that is too acidic will ultimately affect our nutritional status, as the excess acids leech minerals out of our bodily tissues. At the same time, there will be increased elimination via the bowel and kidneys, and also through the skin and sinuses (think mucous) as the body attempts to clear the acidic excess. This is an exhausting metabolic process. (See APPENDIX TWO Acid/alkaline chart.)

MAKE EACH MEAL A NUTRITIONAL OPPORTUNITY

Another serious dietary error is to skip breakfast. The type of breakfast you eat ultimately determines how you will feel throughout the day. Studies have shown that when breakfast is missed the body's metabolic rate remains low for the entire day. Your first meal of the day establishes the amount of sugar in your blood, which translates into how much energy you will have for the day. Your energy level, in turn, determines how you think, act and feel.

This doesn't mean you should stock up on sugary, highly refined and processed breakfast cereals; these will cause the blood sugar to rise rapidly then fall just as rapidly within an hour or so, causing fatigue and hunger. A continued drop in the sugar supply causes fatigue to become exhaustion, with headaches and weakness common. Even when the amount of sugar available to the nerve and brain cells decreases only slightly, thinking becomes slow and confused and nerves tense.

The amount of protein you eat is a key factor in influencing your blood-sugar levels. When there is a combination of carbohydrates (which convert into sugar – the source of energy), protein and fat (which slow digestion), the sugar is gradually absorbed into the blood, maintaining energy at a high level for many hours. However, the typical Australian breakfast of cereal and toast quickly converts into sugar during digestion. When refined sugar is added to cereals and stirred into coffee, and jam is spread on toast, large quantities of sugar pour rapidly into the blood. Blood sugar rises, stimulating the pancreas to produce insulin; the insulin, in turn, causes the liver and muscles to withdraw sugar and store it as glycogen or change it into fat to prevent it being lost through urine. Sugar keeps pouring into the blood, stimulating the pancreas to send more insulin; too much sugar is then withdrawn due to the oversupply of insulin, causing typical low blood-sugar symptoms. Ironically, too much sugar defeats the purpose for which sugar is required: to produce energy!

If, however, breakfast has supplied a small amount of carbohydrates and fat, and a moderate amount of protein, digestion takes place much more slowly and sugar trickles into the blood, giving a sustained energy release hour after hour.

So *don't* skip breakfast. It doesn't need to be big, just nutrient-dense.

The ideal breakfast

The best way to start the day without fatigue is to exercise in the morning. No matter how tired you are, I guarantee it will energise you for the day. Just a brisk 20–40 minute walk is sufficient. Follow it up with a breakfast of rolled oats or barley, a couple of tablespoons of seed mix and wheatgerm, some fresh or cooked fruit, a squirt of linseed oil, and a dollop of 'real' yoghurt containing acidophilus and bifidus (sugar-free).

This breakfast is rich in B-group vitamins, magnesium,

zinc, essential fatty acids (EFAs) and fibre; it provides carbohydrates, fat and protein and is low on the glycaemic
index – meaning your blood-sugar levels will remain stable until lunchtime. And, it doesn't take long to prepare
once you're organised.

Needless to say, processed cereals, white bread, muesli
bars, fruit juices and, heaven forbid, greasy cooked break-
fasts are not acceptable! A frightening indication of how
nutrient-empty most processed cereals are was revealed in a
study carried out on puffed wheat. Four groups of rats were
placed on special diets: group one was fed whole wheat,
water and vitamins; group two was fed puffed wheat, water
and vitamins; group three was fed water and sugar; and
group four was given only water and nutrients. Group one
lived for one year; group two lived two weeks; group three
lived four weeks; and group four survived for eight weeks.
It has been suggested that the process of puffing the grains
(they are placed under 1500 lbs per square inch of pressure and then released) may produce toxic changes in the
grain, resulting in a nutritious substance becoming a poi-
sonous one. The lesson being: the less processed the grain,
the better. A whole grain is *always* more nutritious than a
processed one, and generally less expensive. (Compare the
cost of a bag of plain whole oats to a box of any well-known
processed breakfast cereal.) Try not to over-rely on wheat

products as energetically they are considered a 'tiring' grain. Constantly vary your grains. The same principle applies to lunch and dinner.

Before leaving the breakfast table, fill up at least one litre bottle of water and keep it by your side all day. Simple dehydration can often be the cause of tiredness, especially when accompanied by persistent yawning and headaches.

Here are some delicious recipes for you to choose from that will make varying your grains easy.

SEED MIX

Linseeds
Sesame seeds
Sunflower seeds
Pumpkin seeds
Almond meal
Rice bran, barley bran or oat bran

Use equal quantities of the above ingredients. Grind seeds in blender. Mix all ingredients together and refrigerate in an airtight container.

Breakfast serving suggestion
   4 tablespoons seed mix
   1 grated apple
   ½ cup yoghurt

Blend seed mix well with yoghurt, and stir in grated apple.

In winter the seed mix can be added to cooked oats or rice, and eaten with warm stewed fruit and yoghurt.

Swiss-style muesli

~ Serves 4 ~

The grains are best left to soak overnight but even a half-hour soak (put them in water before you shower and dress) will still provide delicious results.

1 cup rolled oats
1 cup barley flakes
1½ cups water
1 apple
1 banana
½ cup sheep's milk yoghurt
2 tablespoons chopped hazelnuts
1 tablespoon chopped almonds
2 tablespoons wheatgerm
1 tablespoon honey
1 cup blackberries, blueberries or cherries
1 tablespoon toasted sesame seeds

Soak oats and barley in the water overnight. Leave apple unpeeled and remove core. Either grate apple and mash banana, or process them in a food processor briefly until chopped. Add to the soaked oats and barley together with all other ingredients and serve.

BREAKFAST RICE
~ *Serves 6* ~

1½ cups raisins (chopped figs are a delicious substitute)
1 tablespoon grated lemon rind
1 cinnamon stick
1½ cups apple or pear juice
5 cups leftover cooked brown rice
½ cup almonds or walnuts, loosely chopped and lightly roasted

Simmer raisins, lemon rind and cinnamon stick in juice for a few minutes, until raisins are plump. Add rice, simmer for a few more minutes, turn off heat, add nuts and let stand for 10 minutes before serving with soy, rice or oat milk.

A few tablespoons of seed mix on top and a dollop of yoghurt are highly recommended.

WHEAT-FREE/YEAST-FREE MUESLI
~ *Serves 6* ~

2 cups organic rolled oats
1 cup oat bran

1 cup barley bran
1 cup barley flakes
½ cup golden linseeds

Mix all ingredients well and keep in an airtight container in the fridge. Serve with fresh fruit and soy or rice milk, or apple and pear juice. Alternatively cook with a small amount of water and eat hot, as a muesli-porridge. This is especially gorgeous with hot soy milk, a dollop of yoghurt and baked plums.

This recipe is a base which you can imaginatively and deliciously add to and enhance; e.g. wheatgerm, lecithin, walnuts, almonds, rice bran etc.

Buckwheat Porridge
~ *Serves 3–4* ~

1 cup raw buckwheat groats (wholegrain)
2 cups water

Bring water to the boil and add buckwheat. Return to the boil and simmer gently until buckwheat is soft but not mushy, and the water is absorbed.

Serve with baked apple and cinnamon, or banana and honey plus the milk substitute of your choice.

Rice porridge

~ *Serves 3—4* ~

1½ cups rice flakes (rolled)
3½ cups water

Place rice flakes and water in a saucepan and bring to the boil, then simmer until flakes are soft. Add more water if necessary. Serve with a sprinkling of seed mix, raisins or chopped dates and banana, and soy or rice milk.

Brown rice cakes

~ *Serves 2* ~

2 free-range, organic egg whites, stiffly beaten
1½ cups cooked brown rice
3 tablespoons linseed meal or ground sunflower seeds

Mix ingredients together. Place spoonfuls of mixture onto a greased pan and flatten with back of spoon. Place in a hot oven and cook on both sides until browned and crisp. Spread with tahini or almond butter, mashed banana or stewed plums, and/or a little maple syrup or honey.

Mid-morning snack

A mid-morning snack should consist of a couple of pieces of fruit in season or a vegetable juice.

Vitality lunch

A lunch that will enhance your energy levels should include a salad or vegetables, a small amount of protein, and fruit. A tuna or egg salad; a hummus and salad sourdough sandwich; a tofu burger and tabouli in pita bread; steamed vegetables, chickpeas and brown rice – these are all easy to prepare or purchase options. Try to concentrate on raw whenever possible: that is, if a salad sandwich is the only option it should be a huge salad, with the bread merely functioning to hold it all together. The vitamin, mineral and enzyme content of raw vegetables is extremely important to human nutrition and digestive wellbeing.

Please, do try to avoid this naturopath's horror of the 'double protein': that means no cheese and ham; no smoked salmon and cream cheese; or, even worse, steak and seafood sandwiches! Animal protein takes time and energy to digest. Don't overwhelm your stomach and your hard-working enzymes with two or more proteins. Keep it as simple as possible: one animal protein at a time. A three-course meal consisting of a seafood cocktail entree, a steak or chicken main, and a cheese platter 'dessert' is a truly stomach-challenging combination.

Also try to incorporate adequate amounts of the essential fatty acids (EFAs) in your daily eating routine. EFAs cannot be made by the body and must be supplied through the diet. Every cell in the body needs EFAs. The brain, in particular, has a high concentration of EFAs that aid the transmission of nerve impulses.

There are two main categories: Omega-3, which is found concentrated in oily fish, such as salmon, mackerel and sardines, as well as in flaxseed, soy-bean and pumpkin-seed oils; and Omega-6, which is found in safflower, sunflower, sesame, soy-bean, canola, mustard and corn oils. More about EFAs later, as they deserve a chapter all to themselves (see CHAPTER FIVE Essential fatty acids).

Mid-afternoon slump

Before looking for a quick-fix snack, which is invariably sugar or caffeine based, think active! The movement of muscles through normal activity is important to blood circulation and many of us who sit down all day start to feel sluggish as our circadian (daily rhythm) patterns slow down after lunch. Tissues can only be fed with the nutrients in food if the blood supply is adequate, and it is exercise which promotes blood flow and oxygenation. Indeed, exercise simultaneously transports oxygen and nutrients to cells and enhances the movement of carbon dioxide and waste products from the tissues into the bloodstream and organs that remove waste from the body. Take a brisk walk at lunchtime, take the stairs rather than the lift or, if you honestly cannot get away from your desk, just clench and relax muscle groups from time to time. Deep breathing at your desk each hour will improve your blood flow and keep up your vitality.

It is 3 p.m. and your brain is totally fatigued. In addition to ensuring that you are well hydrated and that your blood-sugar levels are not too low, try this essential oil pick-me-up. Keep a small bottle in your pocket or drawer.

Brain revival blend

6 drops rosemary oil
3 drops lemon grass oil (or petitgrain oil, if feeling anxious)
2 drops basil oil or peppermint oil
2 teaspoons sweet almond oil

Mix all the oils in a 10 ml bottle. Shake well and leave for 2–3 days to blend.

Place a couple of drops on the pulse points of the wrist or throat and inhale the vapour. Alternatively, place a few drops on a tissue and inhale. The inhaled oil is absorbed into the nasal passages and picked up by the olfactory receptors that pass information to the limbic system of the brain, which is where emotions and memory are controlled.

The essential oils, without the base oil of sweet almond, can also be placed directly in an oil burner and inhaled effortlessly throughout the day. This is a very effective transport system for calming the nerves and stimulating brain cells.

Mid-afternoon snack

Rice cakes topped with a nut spread (not peanut butter!) or avocado; a small handful of either almonds or brazil nuts, or seeds; low-fat yoghurt; a piece of fruit or a vegetable juice.

Dinner

Best dinner choices include a large range of vegetables, both green and orange, and a small serve of protein. Keep red meat to an absolute minimum; instead look to beans, legumes, fish, free-range chicken and soy products (tofu, tempeh, soy beans and miso). The protein component of our diet is a small but important consideration: it is essential in the creation of neurotransmitters, such as dopamine and noradrenalin. If you're not trying to lose weight, add in some complex carbohydrates; consider brown rice, wheat-free pasta, quinoa, wild rice and millet.

For dessert, choose plain yoghurt or fruit, and perhaps a cup of herbal tea or dandelion-root 'coffee'.

Don't prepare any of the above with a microwave. Until further definitive studies are available to us, stick to stir-frying, steaming and baking. It's interesting to note that Dr Bernard Jensen, one of the founders of iridology (the system of iris analysis used by most naturopaths), found that a whole grain cooked in boiling water for an hour will still germinate if planted, whereas a microwave-cooked grain will not. Furthermore, the plastic containers and browning methods used in microwave cooking have all been linked to cancer-forming substances and chemicals. And any part of the body that cannot dissipate heat efficiently or is heat sensitive, such as the lens of the eye or testes, may be damaged by microwave radiation of sufficient power.

CHAPTER FOUR

ESSENTIAL ELIMINATION

I can guarantee, for those of you who have had a naturo-pathic consultation, that you did not escape a fairly intensive scrutiny of your bowel habits. This may have made you feel a little uncomfortable, even possibly made you squirm in your seat, but I can assure you that it is of great relevance to us. We are just as interested in what comes out as well as what goes in. A sluggish bowel creates a sluggish body.

A complete and satisfying morning bowel movement is crucial to healthy energy levels, as a bowel that is over-burdened and backed up prevents the complete absorption of dietary vitamins and minerals. Stagnation of the bowel ultimately rebounds as stagnation of energetics. Optimal colon function, on the other hand, prevents a toxic build-up and ensures appropriate assimilation of nutrients.

The fibre in food is an important bulking agent to the

stool, which aids elimination of waste materials from the colon. Most clients are, understandably, a little indignant when I tactfully but firmly tell them their dietary fibre is inadequate. We need 30–50g of fibre daily. To put this in perspective: three cups of steamed vegetables contains 10g.

I must admit to having a positive enthusiasm for bowel disorders. Watching a constipated client being transformed from a tired, irritated and uncomfortable individual into a radiant, light, unburdened and energetic one is a delight. And this is normally relatively easy to achieve. A high-fibre diet; adequate water consumption of 1½–2 litres daily; sufficient essential fatty acids (EFAs) for lubrication; and regular, brisk exercise are the keys to excellent bowel health.

A liver in good working order is also vital to effective waste elimination. A daily regime of a glass of warm water and lemon juice upon arising, an abundance of bitter greens in the diet and regular cups of dandelion root coffee (always use the roasted dandelion root, rather than the instant lactose-infused dandelion granules) is also bowel-helpful.

BITTER FOODS

Bitter-tasting foods and herbs stimulate liver function and digestion; however, modern eating patterns seem to have almost completely excluded them from our diet. We do have taste buds for bitter foods and they're there for a reason. Don't let them become obsolete!

The average person has about 10 000 taste buds on their tongue, divided between sweet, sour, salty and bitter. I can guarantee that most of us seriously under-utilise the tiny cluster of cells found at the back of the tongue that respond to the bitter taste in food.

An interesting selection of bitter-tasting foods includes:
- endive
- chicory
- silver beet
- rocket
- radicchio
- cos lettuce (outer leaves)
- mustard greens
- watercress
- dandelion leaf
- dandelion root (coffee).

FIBRE FIGURES

Fibre is the part of plant food that is undigested in the small intestine. There are two types of fibre: soluble and insoluble.

Insoluble fibre increases stool bulk, and so speeds up transit time and promotes regular bowel health. The best sources of insoluble fibre are wheat and rice bran, legumes, nuts, seeds, and the skins of fruit and vegetables. Soluble fibre lowers serum cholesterol by binding cholesterol-containing bile acids and cholesterol, and preventing them from being absorbed. It forms a gel when mixed with liquid, hence its name. Soluble fibre is found in fruits and vegetables, oat and barley bran, dried beans and peas, flax seed and psyllium husks.

Dietary fibre is not substantially broken down by digestive enzymes. Once it reaches the large intestine it undergoes a bacterial fermentation process, which produces short chain fatty acids (SCFA). These SCFAs nourish bowel cells, influence the way in which the body uses cholesterol and affect the utilisation of blood sugars. Dietary fibre slows the digestive process, thereby producing a slow release of nutrients into the bloodstream.

Fibre-rich foods also contribute to satiety; their bulk fills the stomach and they take longer to eat due to the amount of chewing required. A dramatic increase in dietary fibre may initially cause some flatulence and discomfort due to the gut fermentation of plant fibres and bran; however, if the increase is gradual this should not occur. Aim for 30–50 g fibre daily (see APPENDIX THREE for examples of foods containing 10 g fibre).

Stella, nine years old, was a very sick little girl when she came along to see me. She was significantly undernourished, had pale blue circles under her eyes and found it difficult to climb the stairs to my rooms. She had very little in the way of energy reserves. She had a history of chronic constipation and headaches, intermittent severe abdominal pain and lassitude. Stella had been hospitalised twice with severe bowel impaction. The gastroenterologist she had seen placed her on a regime of fairly strong laxatives.

Despite her poor health she was a bright young girl with a charming, sunny personality and a gentle nature. After taking a comprehensive health history, which included an iris analysis and an examination of her nails and tongue, and eliminating any possible physical causes of Stella's constipation, I then went through her diet with a fine toothcomb.

Stella's favourite foods were white bread, milk and cheese – all rather fibreless and constipating foods. Although initially her mother wasn't keen to eliminate milk, we gradually reduced Stella's consumption; replaced white toast with porridge and linseed meal; found a wholemeal bread she liked; increased her intake of fruits and vegetables; and ensured she was having adequate essential fatty acids by adding a metric teaspoon of flaxseed oil to her porridge. I also prescribed some herbs to relax the bowel and prevent muscular spasm, plus calcium and magnesium.

Stella was very compliant and, after a few hiccups, we eventually achieved a constipation-free zone for her. I should add, we also ran some blood tests for food allergies that confirmed she was allergic to brewer's yeast and baker's yeast; cow's, goat's and sheep's milk; and egg white. Stella's energy picked up significantly, her headaches disappeared and she lost the pale blue circles from beneath her eyes. Over a period of months she gradually put on weight and regained a healthy tone to her skin. She also shot up. At a recent four-month review I barely recognised her; she was at least 8 cm taller and positively glowing with good health.

CHAPTER FIVE

ESSENTIAL FATTY ACIDS

In chapter three when we discussed the importance of essential fatty acids (EFAs) in the diet, I mentioned that EFAs are found concentrated in the brain and aid in the transmission of nerve impulses. Let's tease this out a bit further.

TYPES OF ESSENTIAL FATTY ACIDS

EFAs can be divided into two main groups: Omega-3 and Omega-6. Omega-3 (alpha-linolenic acid) is found in marine fish oils (EPA) and flaxseed oil, as well as in pumpkin seed oil, soy-bean oil, canola and mustard seed oils. A widely recognised source of Omega-6 (linoleic acid) is evening primrose oil (EPO); sesame oil, sunflower oil, safflower oil, walnut and canola oils are also good sources. There is a smaller, third group known as the Omega-9 fatty acids; these have similar benefits to Omega-3 and are found in olive, avocado, hazelnut, almond and soybean oils. These are collectively called essential fats: they must be obtained through our diet as our bodies cannot make or synthesise them. They are similar to vitamins; in fact, they were once called vitamin F.

CHARACTERISTICS

All groups of fatty acids are crucial to a fully functional brain. Recently, EFAs have attracted much attention for their role in infant brain development, attention deficit disorder (ADD) and dyslexia. They are required for brain development and adult brain function, having a positive effect on learning and behaviour as well as vision. The brain is the organ richest in essential fats. EFAs in the brain elevate mood and lift depression, which is one of the reasons why EPO is used so successfully in treating PMS and postnatal depression.

EFAs are also components of nerve cells, cellular membranes and hormone-like substances called prostaglandins. Prostaglandins affect the way hormones act upon cells, but do not behave as hormones themselves. They're involved in many physiological processes, such as blood supply, smooth muscle contraction, nerve transmission, water retention, electrolyte balances and blood clotting.

Essential fats assist the body to produce energy. It

has recently been postulated that an imbalance in EFA metabolism may explain the disruption to the immune system, so frequently observed in chronic fatigue syndrome (CFS). Indeed, a controlled trial with CFS sufferers demonstrated a significant reduction of symptoms when they took EFAs (EPO and fish oil).

In addition, EFAs have anti-viral properties. Studies show that natural-killer cell activity (lymphoid cells that attack abnormal cells) can be moderately increased with EPO, and significantly increased with fish oil. These EFAs remove cholesterol from the viral envelope (membrane surrounding the virus-infected cell), preventing viral replication.

Every cell in our body is surrounded by a membrane composed of EFAs and high-density lipoproteins, that is, good cholesterol. This double-layer membrane is selectively permeable, allowing only certain vitamins and minerals to enter and exit the cell. It also forms a defence against unwanted visitors, such as food particles, certain toxins and bacteria. This outer membrane requires good-quality EFAs, on a daily basis, to form healthy, flexible cell walls.

EFAs are further required to transport minerals and assist in their metabolism. An added bonus of regularly including EFAs into our diets is that they increase our metabolic rate. That means we burn up calories faster – not such a bad side effect!

DEFICIENCY – SIGNS AND SYMPTOMS

If we consider that one of the major roles of dietary EFAs is in the formation of a secure cell membrane, then a deficiency must have a significant impact. A diet low in Omega-3 and Omega-6 EFAs is sure to result in a poor-quality cell membrane and possible disruption to the everyday 'ins and outs' of normal cell function. A weakened cell membrane, for example, will cause a diffusion of magnesium (largely an intracellular mineral) out of the cell and into the extracellular environment. The loss of key nutrients will impair the metabolic machinery of the cell, and ultimately affect energy levels. No point putting the right ingredients in, only to find they slip right out again! Compromised cell walls can lead to potentially devastating consequences: cells, organs and tissues (including skin and hair) can all become damaged, both structurally and functionally.

Given the importance of EFAs to the cellular membrane, you will appreciate how crucial these fatty acids are to effective mitochondria – the power source of each cell. It is here that units of energy, adenosine triphosphate (ATP), are manufactured. I spent many long hours in my early days as a naturopathic student anxiously peering into the inner workings of the cell, and I still have visions of a small group of highly efficient workers, sleeves rolled up, sweating and toiling in the engine room of the mitochondria, shovelling heavy spadefuls of magnesium, coenzyme Q10 and B-group vitamins into a fiery furnace. (The dryness of Anatomy & Physiology 101 required a little imaginative input to lighten the study load. Sad, I know, but an improvement on my frequent teary outbursts in Biochemistry 101 when confronted with the Krebs Cycle!)

A mitochondrial dysfunction can result in weakness; fatigue; central-nervous-system disorders, such as stroke, dementia and Parkinson's disease; as well as a whole host of other disorders, including pancreatic and liver dysfunction, and renal and colonic disorders. Therefore, as well as providing the essential base nutrients for the production of cellular ATP, we also need to consider the state of the outer cell membrane.

GETTING THE BLEND RIGHT

The most concentrated form of EFAs are found in certain seeds and nuts (EFAs in a shell, so to speak), as well as cold-water fish and flaxseed oil. Remember, however, that we need a ratio of approximately 2:1 of Omega-3 to

Omega-6. This means combining a diet of high-fat, cold-water fish, and flaxseed, soy bean and pumpkin seed oils, with smaller amounts of safflower, sunflower, canola and walnut oils.

Another way of ensuring adequate dietary intake of Omega-6 would be to regularly consume a seed and nut mix containing fresh sunflower and sesame seeds and walnuts; plus 1–2 tablespoons daily of a well-balanced flaxseed oil blend for Omega-3. (See APPENDIX FOUR for a comprehensive list of the Omega-3 content of seafood, plus some recipes.)

NEVER heat an EFA. Oils that have been heated or, for that matter, subjected to the destructive effects of light and oxygen result in a toxic chemical mess – trans-fatty acids. Consume your oils cold from dark glass bottles.

CHAPTER SIX

DIGESTIVE DISORDERS
AND EXHAUSTION

FOOD ALLERGIES

Food allergies are more common than you think. One day I am going to write a book on the advisability of milk and pineapple consumption for humans, but that's another story. I'll give you a hint. I regularly send clients, with the appropriate symptoms, for a blood test to determine if they have any food allergies. This is not a scratch test or a Vega-machine analysis, but a scientific, biochemical method of challenging blood against over ninety different foods for an IgG reaction – that is, an antibody is formed against a particular food. In the years I have been in practice, 98 per cent of food allergy tests come back positive to dairy, pineapple and the cola nut; closely followed by yeast and wheat. This tells us something.

Ponder this for a moment, although humans have

been drinking milk since 4000 BC, the milk we consume today is a far cry from the 'real' thing of the past. Today's milk is loaded with antibiotic residues to combat mastitis and other diseases in cows; plus various pesticides and herbicides that enter the milk through the bovine food chain; and, to add to this far from appetising cocktail, there are traces of detergent from the milking equipment. The whole lot is then pasteurised, killing not only bacteria and TB bacilli but also, alas, all the crucial enzymes and helpful bacteria that render it digestible. Vitamins are lost and the milk proteins are structurally altered so that whatever remains is hard for the body to digest and assimilate. Hardly a healthy drink!

Cravings

People with undiagnosed and unmanaged food allergies or intolerances feel unwell much of the time, and, therefore, may never associate their health problems with the offending foods. Indeed, I often find that clients with food allergies or intolerances crave the very foods to which they are intolerant. Endorphins are commonly released after ingesting the allergic food, which in turn stimulate the 'pleasure-reward' area of the brain. In order to prolong or repeat this pleasurable sensation we continue to consume the foods responsible for eliciting this response.

This connection between food allergy and addiction is most often seen with wheat and dairy allergy – the foods most commonly known to elicit an adverse response.

Signs and symptoms of food allergies

Food allergies can be seriously debilitating. Symptoms include: bloating, alternating constipation and diarrhoea, abdominal pain, sinusitis, post-nasal drip, joint pain, eczema, fluid retention, dark circles under the eyes, frequent urination and excessive thirst. In addition, symptoms associated with food allergies, or other adverse reactions to food, specific to the brain and nervous system include: dizziness, poor concentration, insomnia, mental exhaustion, irritability, headache, and resistant and recurring fatigue. Just one of these symptoms is physiologically tiring but a collection of them is positively exhausting.

The absorption of nutrients from food is affected due to gut permeability and irritation, which so often goes hand in hand with food allergy; and the dietary intake of many nutrients is also frequently restricted due simply to avoidance of large food groups.

Julia was referred to me by her doctor who after exhaustive testing was at a loss to explain her stomach cramps and abdominal bloating. Julia suffered from frequent and excruciating stomach pain that was normally accompanied with diarrhoea, especially after breakfast. When she was cramp free, however, she was often constipated, sometimes skipping a few days without a bowel movement.

At only twenty-seven years of age, Julia was finding it increasingly difficult to get out of bed in the mornings, despite having sufficient sleep. This was particularly frustrating as she loved her job and was a highly motivated young woman. She had also gained approximately 4 kg in weight over the past couple of years, despite a relatively stable lifestyle and diet. Before eliminating any foods from Julia's diet, I asked her to keep a diet diary for me throughout the next week and to make a note beside the meals that caused any of the symptoms she had reported experiencing. I strongly suspected a dairy allergy since cramping and diarrhoea are common symptoms.*

Julia had travelled to Africa and Turkey in the past, so to rule out any intestinal parasitic infection we arranged with her doctor to do a stool analysis. Fortunately these investigations returned a negative result.

After we sat down and went through Julia's diet diary some obvious conclusions could be drawn: ice-cream, hot chocolate and cake normally resulted in abdominal pain and bloating; as did cappuccinos and melting moments (cream biscuits). However, there was also pain and discomfort associated with relatively benign meals, such as salads and coleslaw, and with meals involving chilli and garlic. Julia was getting married shortly and was keen to have her health problems totally resolved by the wedding day, so we ordered a blood test for food allergies.

The lab report revealed allergies to cow's milk (a very strong positive), brewer's yeast (a reasonably strong positive), and to barley, wheat and cola nut (mild reactions). I suspected the pain Julia experienced when consuming raw vegetables and certain spices was due to a worn and damaged intestinal mucosa. This had probably been caused by years of eating foods she was unknowingly allergic to, resulting in a mild, but chronic, inflammatory state in the intestines that gradually wore away the protective mucosal lining. Eating raw vegetables too quickly, without chewing sufficiently, will also cause some abdominal pain and bloating due to an inadequate break down of carbohydrates resulting in fermentation and gas.

Within weeks of eliminating the offending foods and commencing some serious gut repair Julia's bowel returned to normal; the stomach cramping virtually disappeared and she lost weight (food allergies often cause fluid retention). Her wedding day was perfect; no painful and dress-tightening lower-abdominal bloating, and no stomach discomfort.

Due to her cow's milk intolerance, Julia needs to pay special attention to include adequate calcium in her diet, especially as there is a family history of osteoporosis. So she makes a concerted effort to regularly consume fish with bones (e.g. tinned salmon and sardines), almonds, broccoli and green leafy vegetables, and unhulled tahini. A small and delicious price to pay for a pain-free abdominal region.

Note: Symptoms of cow's milk allergy include: multiple digestive disorders, such as diarrhoea, constipation, vomiting, abdominal pains, cramps, bloating, colic and gas; recurring urinary tract infections; catarrhal build-up in the ears, nose, throat, vagina, bowels and lungs;

asthma; runny nose; skin rashes and eczema; lethargy, irritability and blue circles below the eyes (remember Stella). See APPENDIX FIVE *for a guide to Non-dairy calcium sources.*

Allergy detection

If you suspect you may have a food allergy there are a few simple measures you can take at home to check if this is the case.

Pulse testing

For this test you need to abstain from a particular food for at least a few days, but preferably a month. Before eating the same food again, take your pulse at rest, counting beats per minute. Then eat the food by itself, and take your pulse again at rest after five minutes and then ten minutes later. If your pulse is elevated by more than ten beats per minute, this indicates a strong likelihood of food allergy or intolerance. (Food allergies may cause the release of the stress hormone adrenalin, which usually causes a rise in the pulse rate.) Pulse testing is not time consuming, can be performed in the privacy of your own home, and is remarkably accurate and very inexpensive.

Food challenging

Another exercise you can do at home is the elimination and challenge test.

You will need to avoid the suspected food for six weeks. This means total avoidance: not one iota of the offending food is permitted, then reintroduce the food after a six-week exclusion. If allergic, your symptoms should return within the first twenty-four hours of consuming the suspected food.

The standard elimination test

Part one: elimination of common allergens

If you suspect food allergies may be causing or contributing to your fatigue but you cannot clearly identify the culprit or culprits, the best course of action is an elimination test where a standard group of suspect foods are eliminated over a four- to eight-week period. One food from each excluded group is challenged; a diet and symptom diary is kept and problem foods are clearly identified. Foods to avoid include dairy, wheat, yeast, eggs, corn, soy, peanuts, oranges, tomato, food additives, coffee, alcohol, oils and fats (except the EFAs). Before you throw your hands up in horror and, in a trembling tone, mutter, 'But what is left to eat?' remain calm, plenty of options are left!

All fruits except tomatoes and oranges; all vegetables; most proteins, including meat, poultry, fish, beans/legumes (except soy); all nuts, except peanuts; all seeds; all grains except wheat or corn. Permitted grains would include oats, rice, millet, barley, rye, quinoa and amaranth. If you wish to test an allergy to gluten, you will need to strike oats, rye and barley off the list for a short while as well. (Gluten-containing grains include wheat, rye, barley and oats.) Seeing that you are already eliminating wheat and corn, what's another three grains? Keep in mind that bulgar, couscous, spelt and kamut, being wheat-derived or wheat-related, also contain gluten.

Refer to the menu suggestions in APPENDIX SIX Elimination diet menu plans to help you make these restrictions 'do-able'. Being mentally prepared to make this commitment is important, but just as important is to be prepared in the kitchen. Take time before commencing to plan your elimination diet food options: read through a few inspiring allergy-free cookbooks and stock the kitchen cupboard with an interesting range of permitted foods.

Part two: challenge diary
The food challenge process occurs once the elimination diet has been adhered to for at least four weeks. Eat only one of the restricted foods throughout a particular day; in conjunction, of course, with all your allowable foods. Eat the challenged food at breakfast, lunch and dinner. Keep careful records of the foods eaten and note in a diet diary all

symptoms observed (see APPENDIX SEVEN for a Food challenge diary you can photocopy and use). Food challenges occur for one day and symptoms are noted for that day as well as the next day. Following a food challenge, the challenged food is withdrawn until all other foods are challenged, even if no adverse symptoms were noted. A full day should elapse before another food is challenged. As well as recording symptoms, you may also wish to perform the pulse test, discussed previously, after the challenged food is eaten.

GUT PERMEABILITY— ALSO KNOWN AS 'LEAKY GUT'

The gut wall – our safety blanket

The small intestine acts as a barrier to toxic compounds and macro-molecules. A healthy gut wall made up of a strong, viable mucosal membrane will protect us from dietary bi-products, bacteria and other microbes. The mucosa is the lining of the digestive tract and consists of cellular tissue resting upon a layer of loose connective tissue. In the small intestine the mucosa is formed into folds, which vastly increase its surface area for digestion and absorption.

Causes of gut permeability

We can wear away the lining of our gut mucosa by a variety of means: aspirin, alcohol, stress, dietary deficiencies, drugs (especially the non-steroidal anti-inflammatory drugs), parasitic infection, food allergies and chemotherapy. (I always prescribe glutamine to my clients undergoing chemotherapy. As well as protecting the gut lining, it also helps to decrease the possibility of nausea and mouth ulceration.)

A constant barrage of consuming foods we are allergic to, washed down with a couple of cups of coffee or a few glasses of wine, together with the occasional period of stress and anxiety, will certainly guarantee a gut lining that is worn away and overly porous. Chronic stress can induce dysfunction of the intestinal wall in the ileum (the final portion of the small intestine) and colon by decreasing the protective mucus, increasing membrane permeability and altering the cells of this delicate lining. This in turn allows small food particles to diffuse through the intestinal wall and enter the bloodstream, creating a rather unhealthy situation that ultimately results in a very fatigued and uncomfortable individual.

Signs and symptoms of gut permeability

Symptoms produced by intestinal permeability may be experienced either solely in the abdomen or throughout the whole body. Symptoms include fatigue, malaise, abdominal discomfort and bloating, joint or muscle pain, headache and skin eruptions. Penetration of the gut wall by unwanted substances can result in pathological changes to distant organs and tissues. Certain clinical conditions are strongly associated with altered intestinal permeability; these include the inflammatory bowel diseases, such as Crohn's disease and ulcerative colitis; irritable bowel syndrome; coeliac disease; arthritis; skin conditions, such as eczema and psoriasis; autism; migraines and headache; and chronic fatigue syndrome.

Healing a porous intestine

There is a simple test you can do if you suspect you have a leaky gut, which involves drinking a sugary substance and collecting your urine for six hours thereafter. This method of measuring gut permeability was established by Claude Andre, a leading French researcher in this field. By ingesting two innocuous sugars, lactulose and mannitol, and monitoring their excretion in the urine over a six-hour period, we are able to determine the extent or presence of a permeable gut mucosa. These sugars are not metabolised by humans and the amount absorbed is fully excreted in the urine within six hours. This will give a definitive result – better to know than not to know.

A leaky gut is very easy to heal. I usually use the amino acid glutamine, which has a natural affinity for the gut mucosa, and frequently combine it with aloe vera, slippery elm and liquorice root. All of which have gentle soothing properties designed to ensure a renewed, tightly-sealed, healthy gut wall.

Raw cabbage juice is also a very effective and simple way to treat inflamed gastric mucosa and heal a leaky gut. It is also useful for people suffering from Crohn's disease, ulcerative colitis and gastric ulcers. Two glasses of cabbage juice daily will usually do the trick, and it is not unpleasant! The exact mechanism involved in the healing effect of cabbage juice is not entirely understood; however, glutamine has been identified as one of its major components.

At the same time as taking supplements to heal a leaky gut, a diet low in potential or actual allergens is recommended so further inflammation is not caused. Healing can take anywhere from six weeks to six months, depending on the severity of the damage. It is also important that a good-quality anti-oxidant is taken at the same time because a depletion of the protective compound glutathione is common in leaky-gut syndromes, often contributing to poor liver function. The most effective way to raise liver levels of glutathione is to administer its precursors, cysteine and methionine. These amino acids are the base substances our body uses to make our own internal glutathione and are often common components of a quality anti-oxidant.

Glen, aged forty-five, came to see me with chronic lethargy, recurrent mouth ulcers, depression and, rather alarmingly, a poor memory that was getting progressively worse. He instinctively felt that every time he ate ice-cream his depression and tiredness were exacerbated, and wheat seemed to constipate him. He had been through a battery of tests at a major hospital that were unable to determine the cause of his poor health, and he had also seen an allergy specialist. Glen was emotionally vulnerable and quite anxious. He was frequently bloated and constipated, and suffered from constant headaches. His diet, in an attempt to eliminate possible causes, had become almost unbearably restrictive. Glen had been involved with a poetry group but had to stop participating in live readings due to a frustrating inability to recite by heart. Needless to say, he was, understandably, at the end of his tether.

I immediately requested a blood test for food allergies and coeliac disease (intolerance to the gluten protein found in wheat, barley, rye, oats and triticale), and while waiting for the results started Greg on a regime of glutamine supplementation to repair what I suspected was a leaky gut – this would have the added benefit of improving memory recall. (Glutamine can penetrate the blood–brain barrier and is used as brain fuel; see CHAPTER EIGHT for further details.)

I prescribed a strong-dose vitamin B complex to support the nervous system and some pancreatic enzymes to assist his digestion. The blood tests for food allergies showed that Greg had allergies to durum wheat (also known as hard wheat, durum wheat has more protein than normal wheat and for this reason is used to make pasta), wheat, cow's milk (a very strong positive), egg white, egg yolk and almond. So his gut instinct, if you will pardon the pun, was spot on. His blood tests for coeliac disease returned a positive for gliadin IgA antibodies, so we arranged for Glen to undergo a small bowel biopsy to confirm a diagnosis of coeliac disease. We suspected this was not the case as his food-allergy test had not revealed allergies to any grains except wheat.

Within two weeks of eliminating the allergenic foods, increasing the fibre component of his diet and religiously taking the glutamine there was a discernable improvement in Glen's health. His skin colour improved, losing its pale waxiness; his bowel movements became far more consistent and regular; and Glen remarked that he felt clearer in the head, 'less fuzzy'. After eight weeks his memory began to improve and there was no sign of mouth ulcers. Fortunately, his bowel biopsy did not return a positive for coeliac disease, so the only grain Glen needed to totally eliminate was wheat.

Due to the long-term nature of Glen's illness and a very long-term consumption of allergic foods, we went ahead and ordered a gut-permeability test that did, indeed, reveal a very leaky gut. I replaced the straight glutamine with a glutamine, liquorice root and aloe-vera extract formula to enhance the gut repair and I asked Glen to take it with a quarter of a cup of aloe-vera juice morning and night. Not only would this assist with the mucosal repair, it also treated his constipation. After about three months of treatment, Glen was bounding energetically up the stairs to the clinic, waking refreshed in the mornings with sufficient energy to sustain him throughout the day, his depression had disappeared and he no longer suffered from constipation.

The gut–brain connection

Glen had noted a definite relationship between brain fogginess and dairy consumption; this is certainly not an isolated observation. Many clients commonly report feeling a cloudiness in the head – an inability to think clearly or to concentrate – when there is an excessive consumption of some foods, particularly dairy. And it's not their imagination.

The gastrointestinal tract has an enormous influence over the brain. Brain cells are extremely sensitive to toxic elements and stress, and they must endure our dietary onslaughts and indiscretions for a lifetime.

Opiod peptides are found in foods such as cow's milk and wheat gluten. In certain conditions, such as leaky gut, allergy and EFA deficiency, these peptides have increased access to the brain. Some of these peptides have powerful morphine-like properties and their effect on the brain and nervous system is diverse. A multitude of symptoms may be observed: exhaustion, anxiety, brain fog, irritability, poor memory, aggression, agitation, hyperactivity, insomnia, headache and dizziness. If you notice any of these symptoms after ingesting wheat or dairy, avoid the foods entirely for four to six weeks and then reintroduce them. Avoidance of these foods often results in a clarity and ability to focus not experienced in many years.

CHAPTER SEVEN

VITAMINS AND MINERALS

Having reorganised our diets to ensure maximum energy is derived from each meal through a wise choice of food and the sensible manner in which we consume it, what else can we do to increase energy reserves and combat fatigue?

WHICH NUTRIENTS ARE USED IN ENERGY PRODUCTION?

Bioenergetics is the production of energy at the cellular level. Terms such as the Krebs Cycle, the citric-acid cycle and glycolysis (a series of chemical reactions that produce energy in the cells) may be familiar to you if you have ever had the delightful experience of studying biochemistry. If not, have a look at APPENDIX EIGHT for a non-threatening guide to cellular energy production.

We need to provide the raw materials for our cells and organs to work effectively. Without adequate nutrients, energy production is thwarted and we are unable to fire on all cylinders. The rather forbidding name given to cellular energy is adenosine triphosphate (ATP) and we must produce thirty-two units of it in every cell of our body every minute of the day; ATP is constantly being formed and expended. Key vitamin and mineral deficiencies in our diet result in a decrease in ATP from this optimal requirement. As ATP is central to our understanding of fatigue let's tease this out a bit more.

All of the energy that is extracted from food is converted to ATP: the form in which the body stores energy. In order to release this energy the body converts ATP to a slightly different molecule through a long chain of reactions that are dependent on various vitamins and minerals. To convert dietary protein to energy, for example, we require, at the very least, vitamins B6, B12 and folic acid. Therefore, the importance of obtaining adequate amounts of many nutrients, either from our diet or supplementation, should not be underestimated.

Minor deficiencies of a number of vitamins can contribute significantly to fatigue. For example, just 15 per cent less than the recommended therapeutic dose of thiamine pyrophosphate, an important component of vitamin B1, can lead to symptoms of irritability, mild depression and slight fatigue. A 25 per cent deficiency of thiamine pyrophosphate can result in Wernike-Korsakoff syndrome. The major symptoms of this syndrome are poor short-term memory, disorientation, jerky eye movements, ataxia (staggering gait) and, in its chronic state, brain damage.

Let's look at some of these individual nutrients and assess their importance in energy production. Please note that each of these vitamins and minerals could also be discussed in terms of their impact on other body systems, such as the gastro-intestinal tract, skin or hormone production, but since the scope of this discussion is fatigue we shall keep our focus on these nutrients and their role in energy production. Bear in mind, however, that all body systems are interdependent and the effect of taking supplements for any one system, in this case energy production, will impact positively on many other systems.

A beautiful example of this is the wide-ranging impact of coenzyme Q10. By taking therapeutic amounts of CoQ10 (see page 104) to overcome our fatigue, not only do we manufacture more units of ATP, but we also protect our heart muscle, increase our anti-oxidant status, protect against periodontal disease, boost our immune system and help prevent oxidative damage to our brain.

Therefore, the fantastic positive effects of using nutritional supplements to overcome, in this instance fatigue, also have extensive cross-over benefits to many other body systems.

THERAPEUTIC DOSES TO INCREASE ENERGY PRODUCTION

'Recommended therapeutic dose' vs 'Recommended daily allowance'

Throughout REVIVE, I provide the recommended therapeutic dose (RTD) of vitamins and minerals, not the recommended daily allowance (RDA).

The RDA (also known as the recommended daily intake, RDI) is based on the minimum amount required to prevent short-term-deficiency disease, rather than the prevention of chronic disease and achievement of optimum health. It does not take into account the nutritional content of our food or individual factors. For example, the RDA for vitamin C in Australia is 40 mg daily for men and 30 mg daily for women. The consumption of food containing this amount of vitamin C should prevent scurvy, but in particular situations this amount would be insufficient. For instance, plants grown in areas where the soil quality is poor will have a significantly reduced vitamin C content; or in conditions such as bowel disease where absorption of nutrients is detrimentally affected, individual requirements of vitamin C will be much greater than the RDA. (Not to mention smokers, who need an additional 30 mg of vitamin C per cigarette!)

The RTD, however, is based on achieving a therapeutic outcome. It is now widely recognised that the long-term, inadequate intake of many nutrients results in chronic diseases that may take years to manifest. Nutritional requirements necessary to prevent chronic diseases are higher than those required to prevent the effects of short-term-deficiency conditions. In the last twenty years there has been much evidence that shows nutrients at doses far beyond the RDA act as therapeutic agents in the body, and are able to effect positive change. Vitamin C, for example, taken at an hourly dose of 500–1000 mg significantly reduces the severity and duration of the common cold.

B-group vitamins

The B-group vitamins help maintain the health of the nerves, skin, eyes, hair and liver; as well as healthy muscle tone in the gastro-intestinal tract and effective brain function. They are coenzymes involved in energy production, and are useful in alleviating fatigue, depression, anxiety and insomnia. There are thirteen B-group vitamins, the most commonly prescribed being vitamins B1, B2, B3, B5, B6, B12, folic acid, inositol, biotin and choline. The B-group vitamins are all water soluble and are therefore not stored well in the body, being easily washed away during periods of stress or dieting, and by alcohol, tea and coffee. We need to replenish our stores daily, either with the food we eat or supplementation.

The B-group vitamins should be taken together as their functions are interrelated and they frequently depend on one another to catalyse many chemical reactions. When a greater amount of any one B vitamin is occasionally required to treat a particular disorder, it should be taken with a general B-complex formula to ensure it does not cause a depletion of the others.

Vitamin B1 (Thiamine)
Description
This member of the B-complex group is involved in the production of energy at a cellular level; therefore, even minute deficiencies can result in fatigue and anxiety. The body stores very little in the way of vitamin B1 and a deficiency can occur within a few weeks if intake is reduced. Vitamin B1 is found mainly in skeletal muscle, heart muscle, brain and liver. It optimises cognitive activity and brain function and has a positive effect on growth, energy

and learning capacity. It also acts as an anti-oxidant, protecting the body against the degenerative effects of ageing, smoking and alcohol consumption.

Deficiency

Low thiamine levels result in poor appetite, nervousness, intestinal disorders, depression, failure to concentrate, constipation, irritability and even sciatica. Quite commonly a thiamine deficiency results in a tingling of the hands and feet, and calf muscles may be particularly tender. In a severe deficiency (often due to alcoholism), mental confusion and a marked deterioration of short-term memory are symptoms.

Antagonists

Tea and coffee destroy vitamin B1; antibiotics, sulpha drugs and the oral contraceptive pill may decrease vitamin B1 levels. A high-carbohydrate diet increases the need for this vitamin, and normal cooking processes almost entirely destroy it. Its absorption from the diet requires the presence of folic acid; therefore, a deficiency of folate may result in a vitamin B1 deficiency.

Sources

Excellent sources include brown rice, egg yolks, legumes, liver, wheatgerm and whole grains. Brussels sprouts, nuts, oatmeal, prunes and raisins are also good sources. (See APPENDIX NINE for a delicious brussels sprout recipe. No sneering, please, this is a much maligned vegetable and a very good source of vitamin B1.)

Recommended therapeutic dose

The RTD is 100 mg three times per day. (Don't worry too much about taking these nutrients separately, as there are various formulas available that can be combined to reduce the number of tablets.)

Vitamin B2 (Riboflavin)

Description

Vitamin B2 is responsible for the conversion of fatty acids for energy production, and is an active constituent of enzymes involved in cellular respiration: a process which ensures each cell uptakes and uses oxygen efficiently. Vitamin B2 alleviates eye fatigue, facilitates the use of oxygen by the tissues of the skin, hair and nails and helps the absorption of iron and vitamin B6. It also regulates thyroid gland function. All very important factors in manufacturing and maintaining appropriate energy levels.

This is the vitamin that turns your urine yellow and it was originally used to treat chelosis (cracks in the corner of the mouth) and keratitis (an inflammatory skin condition).

Deficiency
Common symptoms of low vitamin B2 levels include cracked lips and sore tongue; burning, itching eyes; digestive disorders; hair loss; vaginal itching; and poor immunity. The skin on the face may become red, greasy and scaly, especially at the sides of the nose.

Antagonists
Some antibiotics increase our need for vitamin B2, great losses can occur in foods that are subjected to light or cooked in salt water, and it is dissipated by diarrhoea, liver disease and alcohol. The use of the oral contraceptive pill and strenuous exercise increase our requirement for vitamin B2.

Sources
High levels of vitamin B2 are found in egg yolks, legumes, meat, milk, spinach, whole grains, brewer's yeast and yoghurt.

Recommended therapeutic dose
The RTD is 100 mg three times per day.

Vitamin B3 (niacin, niacinamide, nicotinic acid)
Description

Vitamin B3's main function is to support the nervous system but it is also required for the healthy functioning of the gastrointestinal tract and the skin. Vitamin B3 forms part of the enzymes that play a crucial role in glycolysis – that is, the extraction of energy from carbohydrates and glucose.

It is one of the components of a substance known as Glucose Tolerance Factors (GTF, the other components being chromium and the three amino acids: glycine, cysteine and glutamine acid), which plays an active role in the uptake of insulin and in stabilising blood-sugar levels. Niacin helps regulate appetite and is required for the production of hydrochloric acid, a necessary factor for an efficient digestive system. Indeed, due to its ability to increase energy by improving the uptake of nutrients from food, it is extremely beneficial in treating fatigue, irritability and digestive disorders.

Deficiency

The symptoms of vitamin B3 deficiency vary considerably, but show up on the tongue, skin, and in the gastrointestinal tract. The tongue is often sore, painful and fissured, and can resemble the tread of a car tyre. Many of my clients are surprised when, during a consultation, I ask them to stick their tongue out – not something that most adults are entirely comfortable with. However, much can be discovered during this inspection, not the least of which is a fairly serious B-vitamin deficiency (see APPENDIX TEN Tongue tales, for a detailed description of what the tongue reveals). Vitamin B3 was originally discovered as a cure for pellagra, a dietary deficiency disease characterised by the three Ds: dermatitis, diarrhoea and dementia.

Specific symptoms of inadequate B3 levels include loss of appetite, lassitude, limb pains, dizziness, depression, anxiety and, in the extreme, hysteria and psychotic episodes. (A great deal of work has been done in the treatment of schizophrenia with vitamin B3.)

Antagonists

Fortunately vitamin B3 is a relatively stable vitamin, far more resilient to heat than its other B-group brothers, although the processing of grains can remove up to 80 per cent.

Sources

Niacin is found in beef liver, brewer's yeast, poultry, wheatgerm, whole grains, eggs, fish, cheese and peanuts.

Recommended therapeutic dose

The RTD is 100–300 mg per day.

Caution: A harmless flush sometimes occurs after taking niacin in the form of niacinamide. High doses of niacin should not be taken in pregnancy or in the case of ulcers, diabetes, glaucoma, gallbladder or liver disease

Vitamin B5 (Pantothenic acid)

Description

The most significant factor regarding vitamin B5 and human health is its impact on the adrenal glands. It is for this reason known as the 'anti-stress' vitamin, as hormones produced by the adrenals help to counteract stress. This vitamin assists in converting fats, carbohydrates and proteins into energy; and it supports the auto-immune system, helping to prevent infections.

Vitamin B5 is also involved in the production of key neurotransmitters, such as acetylcholine (important for the nerves) and is needed for the proper functioning of the gastrointestinal tract.

Deficiency

Fatigue and anxiety are the most common symptoms of a vitamin B5 deficiency; headache, nausea and tingling in the hands are often experienced. Low levels of vitamin B5 can cause digestive problems, mainly due to a decrease in hydrochloric acid production (which helps to break down fats and proteins), resulting in symptoms such as gas, bloating, abdominal cramping and discomfort after large meals. This naturally has a big impact on energy production. In animal studies where there has been severe and long-term vitamin B5 deficiency, haemorrhage and destruction of the adrenal glands has occurred.

Antagonists
Food processing and cooking destroys vitamin B5 – more than 50 per cent is lost during the milling of wheat, for example.

Sources
Excellent sources of vitamin B5 include brewer's yeast, eggs, liver, whole wheat, rye, wheatgerm and legumes.

Recommended therapeutic dose
The RTD is 200 mg three times per day.

Vitamin B6 (Pyridoxine)
Description
The discovery of vitamin B6 in the 1930s was, in retrospect, a major breakthrough in the treatment of fatigue-related issues. *The New York Times* reported in 1938 that the discovery of vitamin B6 '. . . which may henceforth be

known as the "vitality vitamin" may account at last for many mysterious conditions in which patients for no known medical reason complain of constant fatigue, listlessness and lack of interest in general.'

Vitamin B6 is crucial to so many body functions that even a minor deficiency can have profound effects on our health. This vitamin is required for the production of adrenal gland hormones and antibodies, helping to support our immune system. Brain chemistry is dependent on vitamin B6, as it is essential for the formation of several neurotransmitters that affect mood, notably serotonin and histamine. Energy production is also dependent on adequate levels of vitamin B6 because it helps to liberate glycogen (stored energy) from the muscles and liver.

Deficiency

Deficiency symptoms include sleepiness, loss of appetite and morning nausea, headache, dizziness, depression, muscular weakness, pains in arms and legs, and irritability. External signs include sore lips and tongue; dermatitis in the area of the nose, behind the ears, corners of the mouth and eyes; and fluid retention, especially of the premenstrual syndrome (PMS) variety.

Antagonists

High-protein diets demand extra vitamin B6. A large hamburger from a fast-food chain, for example, provides approximately, a mere 0.02 mg of B6, while providing a very large quantity of protein. So, in order to metabolise the protein, vitamin B6 must be obtained from another source.

Anti-depressants and all oestrogen therapy, including the oral contraceptive pill, smoking and some food additives increase our need for this vitamin. Diuretics and cortisone drugs block the absorption of vitamin B6; drugs that destroy vitamin B6 include penicillamine, some anti-hypertensive and anti-tuberculotic drugs, and drugs used to treat Parkinson's disease. Cooking reduces or destroys it, while exercise may improve the conversion of vitamin B6 to its more active form in the body.

Sources

Vitamin B6 is found concentrated in brewer's yeast, whole grains, fish, spinach, blackstrap molasses and wheatgerm.

Recommended therapeutic dose

The RTD is 100 mg two to three times per day. An update in 1990 of Cohen and Bendich's 1986 *Review of the Safety of Vitamin B6* indicated that doses of 500 mg or less per day for up to a period of two years were safe.

Vitamin B12 (Cobalamin)
Description
This vitamin is often referred to as the 'energy' vitamin. It rapidly increases energy levels mainly due to its role – together with a number of other vitamins and minerals, such as iron, folic acid, copper, vitamins B6 and C – in the formation of normal red blood cells. It is frequently used to treat pernicious anaemia; in severe cases it is given intramuscularly, one to three times per week, until vitamin B12 stores are replenished.

Vitamin B12 is essential for the health of the entire nervous system; it is involved in the absorption of nutrients and the metabolism of carbohydrates and fats; and it is vital in the production of acetylcholine, a neurotransmitter responsible for memory and learning. It is by far the most potent of all the vitamins – virtually every major aspect of the body's metabolism depends on it, and yet a teaspoon could hold our ration for eight years. Vitamin B12 is a red crystalline substance, and is found in highest concentrations in the liver, heart, brain, kidney, testes, blood, and bone marrow.

Deficiency
Deficiency symptoms, which can often be quite subtle, normally start in the nervous system. Vitamin B12 nourishes

the myelin sheath covering the nerves, which helps maintain the electrical conductivity through the nerves. Early symptoms include tiredness, irritability, decreased attention span, headaches, drowsiness, breathlessness on exertion, ringing in the ears and loss of libido. Weakness of the arms or legs, diminished reflex response, difficulty walking or speaking, or limb jerkiness may also occur.

A vitamin B12 deficiency can cause megaloblastic anaemia, a condition in which red blood cells become enlarged and fewer are formed, leaving the body starved of oxygen, resulting in an anaemic fatigue. This anaemic condition, which is not related to iron deficiency, can lead to a severe deterioration of the spinal cord, brain and peripheral nerves. Psychological symptoms include mood changes and mental slowness, loss of memory and confusion, depression and poor concentration may also result.

Severe pernicious anaemia, a type of megaloblastic anaemia, will cause a red, cracked, sensitive tongue, often ulcerated; and heart palpitations may also be experienced. Long-term deficiency will ultimately result in brain and spinal cord degeneration, causing weakness, numbness, tingling, shooting pains, hallucinations and paranoia.

Antagonists

A vitamin B12 deficiency is commonly due to malabsorption. An enzyme produced by the stomach cells (the 'intrinsic factor') is needed so that B12 (the 'extrinsic factor') can be transported through the intestines and be properly absorbed. Ageing, stress and stomach problems interfere with the body's ability to produce the 'intrinsic factor'.

Hydrochloric acid is also required for the absorption of vitamin B12. At least 22 per cent of the population produces inadequate hydrochloric acid, so although dietary intake of vitamin B12 may be satisfactory, absorption is generally not. A simple but effective way to improve hydrochloric acid production is to sip a glass of water with one teaspoon of apple cider vinegar prior to a meal. (Although, I have a feeling many may prefer an aperitif of Campari and soda?)

Laxatives, overuse of antacids and alcohol all deplete vitamin B12 reserves. Gout medications, anticoagulant drugs and potassium supplements may also block its absorption from the intestinal tract. As this vitamin is found almost exclusively in animal sources, vegetarians are prone to deficiency.

Sources
Vitamin B12 is found in significant amounts only in animal protein foods, including meat, oily fish, egg yolks and dairy products. There are only minute amounts found in tempeh and other fermented soy products; sprouts; mushrooms; and sea vegetables, such as kelp, kombu and nori. Therefore, vegans definitely need to supplement with vitamin B12. The herbs alfalfa, bladderwrack and hops also contain small amounts of this vitamin.

Recommended therapeutic dose
The RTD is 500–1000 mcg per day, and it is best taken in a sustained-release formula or sub-lingually (under the tongue).

So, it should be obvious why I continually emphasise the importance of a good vitamin B complex. This dynamic group of vitamins has an enormous impact on the nervous system, hormone production, synthesis of neurotransmitters and brain function: all factors intimately involved in the treatment of fatigue. While chemically distinct from one another, the B-group vitamins' work in the body is closely related.

How to eat your B-group vitamins

You have probably noticed that many of these key nutrients are found concentrated in brewer's yeast, wheatgerm, molasses, eggs, yoghurt and green leafy vegetables. We really should try to incorporate these foods into our weekly diet. I guarantee that a combination of 1 teaspoon of brewer's yeast mixed into soy milk, or yoghurt, with 1 tablespoon lecithin, wheatgerm and blackstrap molasses will have you sparkling with health and vitality in a week or so, as well as having a visible impact on the health of your hair, skin and nails! If you have a sensitive stomach or are prone to candida you may need to avoid yeast.

THE SPARKLE SHAKE

½ cup apple or pear juice

1 banana

½ cup yoghurt

½ cup soy milk

1 teaspoon blackstrap molasses

1 teaspoon brewer's yeast

1 teaspoon lecithin granules

1 teaspoon wheatgerm

1–2 teaspoons raw honey

⅓ teaspoon kelp powder (optional)

Blend together all the ingredients until smooth. This smoothie can be adapted to suit your own taste. If a particular ingredient in the drink does not appeal or is not well tolerated, avoid it and substitute something more appealing. Other fruits or juices can be used, or no juice and just soy milk. Flavourings such as pure vanilla or almond essence, or a handful of raw almonds or sunflower seeds can be added and blended. Make it work for you.

Let's look at five more nutrients: vitamin C, magnesium, potassium, iron and coenzyme Q10, and assess their role in cellular energy production.

Vitamin C (ascorbic acid)
Description
Vitamin C, also known as ascorbic acid, calcium ascorbate and sodium ascorbate, is most highly concentrated in the adrenal glands, pituitary gland, brain and eye lens. It stimulates adrenal function through the release of adrenalin and noradrenalin, our stress hormones; however, prolonged stress depletes vitamin C in the adrenals and the blood.

Vitamin C also supports our immune response via the production of interferon, a protein produced by cells when challenged by a virus, and helps reduce reactions to food allergies by decreasing the secretion of histamine, a harmful chemical released during an allergic reaction (1000 mg three to four times per day is effective in reducing allergic symptoms).

Vitamin C is, of course, a powerful anti-oxidant and is needed for the metabolism of folic acid and the amino acids tyrosine and tryptophan. Tryptophan is converted in the presence of vitamin C to serotonin, an important brain chemical; serotonin has a relaxing, calming and uplifting effect on the central nervous system. Likewise, the amino acid tyrosine also needs vitamin C to form the hormone adrenalin, which prepares us physiologically to think quickly, run faster and fight harder. Vitamin C, together with glutamine (more about this amino acid later), is also used to treat 'overtraining syndrome', where high levels of physical exertion make an athlete susceptible to infection.

Deficiency

When the body's stores of vitamin C fall significantly, the first sign of deficiency is fatigue. Lowered immunity and poor resistance to infection are also characteristics of inadequate levels of vitamin C; a tendency to bleeding gums and poor wound healing may also be experienced.

Due to its role in adrenal gland function and immune response, vitamin C is especially relevant in the treatment of chronic fatigue syndrome. This condition is characterised by adrenal dysfunction and lowered immunity, with sore throats and swollen or tender glands being common symptoms.

Antagonists

Emotional and environmental stress increases our requirement for vitamin C. Alcohol, analgesics, antidepressants, anticoagulants and steroids reduce levels of vitamin C in the body, and smoking causes a serious depletion (30 mg per cigarette).

Sources

Vitamin C is a water-soluble vitamin and most of our stores of it exit the body within three hours. The body cannot manufacture vitamin C, and it must, therefore, be obtained through diet or supplementation.

The best-known sources of vitamin C are the citrus fruits: oranges, limes, tangerines and grapefruits. The fruits with the highest concentrations are guavas, blackcurrants, rose hips, acerola cherries and kiwifruit, followed by papaya, cantaloupes, oranges, grapefruit and strawberries. Good vegetable sources include red and green peppers, broccoli, brussels sprouts, cauliflower, parsley and dark leafy greens, such as spinach and cabbage. Although there is not much available vitamin C in whole grains, seeds and beans, when these foods are sprouted, their vitamin C content shoots up!

Recommended therapeutic dose

The RTD is 2000–4000 mg in small, frequent, divided doses, including the bioflavonoids. (A constant companion of vitamin C, the bioflavonoids, otherwise known as vitamin P, include rutin, hesperedin, quercitin, catechin and flavones.)

Caution: In pregnancy, the dose should be no more than 500 mg per day. Also take care if combining aspirin and large doses of vitamin C, as this may cause stomach ulceration.

Magnesium
Description

Magnesium is a magnificent mineral. The entire, delicately intricate and complex process of producing energy depends on it. Magnesium is mainly involved in energy production at the Krebs Cycle stage (see APPENDIX EIGHT Cellular energy metabolism), where it plays a major role in turning protein, carbohydrates and fats from our diet into energy. Without sufficient magnesium, an essential ingredient in this cycle is missing and adequate energy simply cannot be produced.

Magnesium not only acts as a catalyst to the breakdown of protein, carbohydrates and fats, it is also responsible for glycogen storage and release, acid/alkaline balance and membrane permeability. A magnesium deficiency can seriously affect other key mineral levels, as it is difficult to maintain adequate body levels of potassium, calcium and sodium unless our magnesium stores are optimal.

Magnesium is perhaps the nutrient most involved in stress. A combination of magnesium deficiency and stress can create a vicious cycle. This is due to the fact that the adrenal glands secrete additional cortisol under stress, which also interferes with magnesium absorption. Even a mild magnesium deficiency predisposes us to stress, which in turn may induce or exacerbate the magnesium deficiency. Certainly stress itself, through the increased release of adrenalin, indicates that magnesium has moved out of the cell, creating a deficiency. Indeed, the results from an interesting trial of athletes taking magnesium are relevant to all stressed individuals. When this group of competition triathletes were given magnesium orotate their swimming, cycling and running times improved; and their serum cortisol and insulin were lowered. In other words, energy production was increased and stress decreased.

Magnesium is a key nutrient used to treat chronic

fatigue syndrome particularly the bone-tiredness experienced by so many chronic fatigue sufferers. It is crucial in enabling muscles to uptake the amino acid creatine. Creatine boosts the growth of lean muscle tissue and enables the muscle to increase its uptake of protein and water, leading to stronger muscles. Creatine is also a vital ingredient of ATP production, yielding energy to muscle cells and enabling us to expand and contract muscles efficiently. Energy from creatine cannot be obtained when a magnesium deficiency exists. Thus, magnesium has a fairly direct role in muscle energetics.

Deficiency

A deficiency in magnesium interferes with the transmission of nerve and muscle impulses. It leads to a hyper-sensitivity to the sensory messages our nerves carry to the brain, causing over-reactions to everyday sensations: the sound of a doorbell becomes so shocking that it makes our hair stand on end and our heart pound or a ticking clock becomes inordinately annoying and intrusive. When magnesium is deficient, we find cells remain in a state of hyper-excitability, unable to return to a normal, calm resting state.

Deficiency symptoms include: muscle weakness and cramping, depression, confusion, insomnia, irritability, noise sensitivity, poor digestion, spasm in the eyelids, pre-menstrual tension (PMS) and rapid heart beat.

Magnesium deficiencies are also at the root of many cardiovascular problems.

Antagonists

The consumption of alcohol, the use of diuretics, diarrhoea, fluoride, profuse sweating, and high levels of zinc and vitamin D increase the body's need for magnesium. Excessive consumption of soft drinks and coffee also decrease our magnesium levels.

Poor insulin production adversely affects our body's cellular stores of magnesium; therefore, those people with diabetes mellitus are particularly susceptible to magnesium deficiency. Cytotoxic and immunosuppressant drugs (commonly used in cancer treatment) may also cause magnesium loss.

In Australia, magnesium levels are often low in the top soil, due to poor land practices and leaching; soil acidity problems reflect an associated decline in magnesium levels. This naturally affects the levels of magnesium in the plants grown in these affected areas. (United States' soils are comparatively lower in magnesium than soils from south-east Australia.)

Sources

Rich sources of magnesium include: grains, such as millet, buckwheat, brown rice, wheat, oats; dark green vegetables (magnesium, a component of chlorophyll, is important in plant photosynthesis); nuts, especially almonds, brazil nuts and cashews; seafood and kelp. Bear in mind, however, that the magnesium content of food will depend on the magnesium levels in the soil where the food is grown.

Recommended therapeutic dose

There are two types of magnesium: magnesium orotate and magnesium aspartate. Magnesium orotate (vitamin B13) transports magnesium into the mitochondria, the power house of the cell where ATP is manufactured.

Magnesium aspartate moves magnesium into the cell fluid, where it improves oxygen utilisation in all muscle tissue and increases creatine uptake. Therefore, by carefully combining the types of magnesium used, we can ensure effective transportation of magnesium for the production of cellular energy.

An appropriate combination would be magnesium aspartate 150 mg three times per day together with magnesium orotate 200 mg three times per day.

Caution: Avoid in cases of severe renal impairment.

Potassium

Description

Potassium is important to normal cell growth and the building of muscle. It is involved in the conversion of glucose to glycogen, which is stored in the liver for future energy needs. Potassium is the primary positive ion found within the cell; it is called an 'electrolyte' because it carries a tiny electrical charge. Potassium combines with sodium to regulate the body's water balance and heart rhythms, and helps to conduct nerve impulses. When the sodium–potassium equilibrium is upset, nerve and muscle functions are detrimentally affected. The part of the brain involved with balance, the cerebellum, is also dependent on adequate levels of potassium.

Deficiency

A potassium deficiency is common, especially with stress, ageing or chronic disease, and fatigue is often the first symptom. Other early symptoms of a deficiency include muscle weakness, restless legs or prickling of the extremities, headache, memory impairment, difficulty concentrating, depression and slow reflexes. Dry skin and an insatiable thirst may also be experienced, and balance may become unstable and physical activity difficult. Low levels of potassium can affect the smooth muscle of the gut, causing gastric cramps, nausea, vomiting and abdominal distension. Long-term, chronic potassium deficiency may result in heart conditions, such as hypertension and cardiac arrhythmia.

Antagonists

Many factors reduce potassium: diarrhoea, vomiting, extreme heat and profuse sweating. Several drugs can also result in hypokalemia (low levels of potassium): diuretics, laxatives, aspirin, digitalis and cortisone. Stress increases the body's potassium requirements, as the secretion of stress hormones causes a decrease in the potassium to sodium ratio.

Sources

Food sources include dates, figs, peaches, bananas, root vegetables (especially potatoes with their skins), leafy green vegetables and blackstrap molasses.

Recommended therapeutic dose

The RTD is 600–1000 mg per day

Caution: Do not take potassium with potassium-sparing diuretics and ACE inhibitors.

POTASSIUM-POWER SOUP

~ Serves 4 ~

This soup has a high-potassium content, mainly due to the potatoes. If you are following a nightshade-free diet, sweet potatoes can be substituted. Avoid potatoes with a green tint; the chemical solanine, which gives the potato its green cast, can interfere with nerve impulses, causing diarrhoea, vomiting and abdominal pain. This potassium soup is a warming nutrient-dense winter drink.

2 potatoes, with skins, roughly chopped
2 cups of chopped vegetables e.g. carrots, celery, celeriac root, parsley,
swedes, parsnips, turnips, beetroot and spinach
ginger or garlic for taste.

Place vegetables in a large saucepan with sufficient water to cover, bring to a gentle boil and then simmer for half an hour. Leave to stand a further 30 minutes, strain and drink hot or cold. It can be refrigerated and kept for 2–3 days, or frozen in individual portions and enjoyed as desired.

To turn this soup into a main meal do not strain, and add either red or brown lentils, mung beans or split green or yellow peas to the base.

Iron

Description

Iron is found in every cell of the body. Its most important function is the production of the haemoglobin molecule, the red blood cell, which supplies oxygen to our tissues, and the myoglobin molecule, which carries oxygen to the muscles. Oxygen starvation occurs as a result of iron deficiency and leads to a general decline in efficiency of the cells. Anaemia is the reduction in the number of red blood cells due to long-term iron deficiency. Ferritin is our stored form of iron.

Iron is also required for a healthy immune system and plays a central role in the production of energy; even a borderline deficiency can cause a noticeable lack of energy. The body contains about 3–4 g iron. Only 8 per cent of our total iron intake is absorbed and actually enters the bloodstream.

Deficiency

One of the commonest signs of an early iron deficiency is waking up tired and generally feeling listless. Exercise may become tiring and muscles can become flaccid. As every organ is dependent upon oxygen, iron loss will affect the lungs, heart, liver, kidneys and skin, leading to more serious problems, such as breathlessness, difficulty swallowing, palpitations after physical exertion, poor vision, dizziness, migraine, insomnia, cramping, slowed mental reactions and even depression.

Iron deficiency is often revealed by skin pallor: the

loss of the healthy pink hue from the nailbeds, or pale rather than the customary pink membranous undersides of the eyelids; cracks at the corner of the mouth may also develop. In more serious cases a tingling in the toes and fingers may be experienced.

Antagonists

Iron deficiency is generally due to insufficient dietary intake. It may also result from intestinal bleeding; poor digestion; excessive menstrual bleeding; a diet too high in phosphorous (e.g. carbonated drinks and red meat); a prolonged use of antacids; excessive coffee or tea consumption (caffeine reduces iron absorption, especially when drunk at mealtimes, and tannins in tea bind iron making it unabsorbable); strenuous exercise, particularly long distance running; and excessive perspiration.

A diet too high in oxalates found in leafy greens, and phytates found in whole grains, can also interfere with iron absorption. Green vegetables, such as spinach, are high in iron but their considerable oxalate content can make this 'green' iron difficult to absorb; and the iron in whole grains, such as wheat and millet, although significant can become bound and insoluble due to the phytates. So, as you can see, choosing a diet adequate in iron is no easy matter.

Enhancing absorption

Although many vegetables and grains contain significant amounts of iron, these take the form of 'non-haems', which are, unfortunately, not readily absorbed through the gut. Meats and fish, however, are high in the 'haem' form of iron and are far easier to absorb. It is estimated that only about 15 per cent of the iron in a typical 'mixed' diet is actually absorbed, and when there is no red meat in the diet this figure drops even further. The vital process of converting non-haem iron to forms that the body can absorb requires vitamin C, so it is essential, particularly for vegetarians, to combine foods containing vitamin C with iron-rich foods in the same meal. Thankfully, in nature iron and vitamin C are often combined – think of a spinach leaf! (See page 87 for a full list of good dietary sources of vitamin C.) Alternatively, taking a vitamin C powder or tablet improves the absorption of iron supplements.

The absorption of iron from a diet that includes meat is about three times that of an exclusively vegetarian diet. The answer, if you are a vegetarian, is to eat an iron-rich diet, consciously loading your diet with exceptionally rich and readily absorbed iron sources, such as blackstrap molasses, watercress, raisins and lentils; and to check your ferritin and iron stores with a yearly blood test. Ideally ferritin stores should be at least 55 nmol/ml (normal range can vary from 10–150 nmol/ml) and haemoglobin should be in the range of 115–165 nmol/ml.

Sources

Rich sources of iron include kelp, blackstrap molasses, wheatgerm, millet, parsley, prunes, red meat, raisins, beetroot and leaves, lentils, dried peaches, dried apricots, dried figs, spinach and oatmeal. For example, 100 g dried peaches provides 4.1 mg iron, 100 g lean beef provides 3.7 mg iron, and blackstrap molasses, for the equivalent weight, yields a very respectable 16.1 mg iron.

Recommended therapeutic dose

The RTD is 15 mg three times per day. Beware of non-organic iron supplements. Never take ferrous sulphate, as it causes constipation and is irritating to the gastrointestinal tract. The best iron tablets to take are in the form of an organic amino acid chelated iron (pronounced 'key-lated'). Ferrous succinate, ferrous fumerate or ferrous aspartate would be wise iron supplement choices. Ferrous fumerate is an especially good choice, because with the help of vitamin C it converts to the very absorbable ferric form of iron. Iron diglycinate, in a chelate form, is especially well-tolerated and will not cause irritation. One of the best assimilated iron supplements available is a liquid iron tonic which uses iron in the form of ferrous lactate in a beetroot and red grape-juice base. It is quickly absorbed, well-tolerated, non-constipating and delicious, and best taken on an empty stomach. When buying an iron supplement always check the label for the type of iron used.

Caution: Only take iron supplements when there is a deficiency as excess iron accumulates in tissues and organs; and do not take when there is an acute infection as bacteria require iron for growth. Ensure that iron supplements are not taken at the same time as zinc and vitamin E supplements, which interfere with iron absorption. If taking the cardiac medication Methyldopa, separate the doses by two hours.

GREEN IRON BOOST — A BLOOD-BUILDING JUICE

1 beetroot with its leaves
3 carrots
½ bunch parsley
1 cup spinach leaves (dark green leaves)

Wash, rinse and dry beetroot leaves, spinach and parsley. Scrub carrots and beetroot well. Alternately feed the ingredients through the juicer, rolling parsley up in the spinach leaves so it feeds through more easily. Drink straight away and slowly – juices should be chewed not gulped!

This truly delicious juice is high in iron, carotenes and chlorophyll, as well as folate, potassium, magnesium and vitamin C.

Helena's first words to me were, 'I'm so tired by three o'clock in the afternoon that I become teary and when I get home from work I find myself snapping at my eldest daughter. No matter how much sleep I get, I still wake up un-refreshed and am finding it increasingly difficult to get out of bed in the mornings. Every day feels like a Monday morning.'

Helena is thirty-five years old, works full-time, and has two daughters aged three and nine. As well as being chronically tired, she had also been having a heavy period every two weeks for the past twelve months. Her face was pale without a hint of pink, and when I examined her fingernails and palms I found pale nail beds and palms without the characteristic red lines. Her tongue was unnaturally flat and looked sore and red. Helena had a previous history of anaemia and, even though she had been taking iron supplements on an occasional basis for the past few years, I suspected an iron deficiency and ordered some blood tests. I also requested an intestinal permeability test to check whether her absorption was possibly compromised. While we waited for the results, I started Helena on an iron-rich diet with an abundance of greens, blackstrap molasses and lentils; and, since she had no objection to red meat, I suggested she include red meat in her diet at least twice weekly. I also rather firmly asked her to increase her water consumption, which was currently stuck in the rather poor 'two-glasses-if-I'm-lucky' regime. Not unusual!

Helena's blood tests confirmed anaemia: both her iron levels and ferritin stores were low. I questioned her about the iron supplements she had been taking and discovered they were a diverse group. The most recent supplement she had used was a liquid iron with a mixture of herbs and yeast. Prior to this she had taken a ferrous sulphate tablet recommended by her doctor which had resulted in constipation and blackening of the stools. This form of iron binds up the bowels and, being inorganic, it is also very poorly absorbed. Beware of this type of iron tablet!

I started Helena on a chelated form of iron to be taken with a vitamin C supplement, or a glass of cherry or grapefruit juice; a vitamin E supplement to protect her red blood cells from the toxic effects of free radicals (to be taken at a different time to the iron supplement); a good-quality vitamin-B complex, to provide adequate vitamin B12 and folic acid, and herbal medicine to assist with her heavy, frequent menses. In addition, Helena agreed to a new dietary regime of starting each day with a large tablespoon of fresh wheatgerm on her muesli at breakfast, and finishing each day with an equally generous spoon of non-sulphured blackstrap molasses.

Helena's gut permeability tests showed a leaky gut and malabsorption. This explained why she continued to be anaemic despite the occasional iron tonic. I therefore started her on a gut-repair program, which simply meant taking a powdered mixture of glutamine, slippery elm, aloe-vera extract and apple pectin. This would, in a friendly fashion, cling to the mucosal walls of the gut, healing any inflammation and repairing worn away and porous mucous membranes. (Glutamine is an essential nutrient for the rapidly dividing cells lining the gastrointestinal tract.) Within four months Helena's blood tests came back with a large elephant stamp. Her iron stores had risen to a far more respectable level, her energy had improved dramatically, she no longer felt depressed or irritable, and her periods had returned to a twenty-four to twenty-six day cycle.

As soon as Helena's iron and ferritin stores showed signs of stabilising we discontinued the iron supplements, and maintained her levels through a suitable diet. Before completing our treatment, I requested a repeat of the gut-permeability test to confirm her gut was positively repaired and to be confident she was well and truly absorbing all the nutrients from her diet. I am happy to report, Helena's test came back with perfect results.

Coenzyme Q10 (ubiquinone)
Description
Coenzyme Q10 (CoQ10) is a vitamin-like substance that plays a crucial role in the production of cellular energy. The main function of CoQ10 is the manufacture of adenosine triphosphate (ATP), which is the basic energy molecule of cells. The amount of CoQ10 present in our cells declines with age.

CoQ10 is a major anti-oxidant and assists heart function by enhancing pumping action and electrical function, as well as lowering blood pressure; it has a mild effect on the metabolic rate and is an immune stimulant. It also improves skeletal muscle; the blood and leg muscle content of CoQ10 is often low in chronic fatigue syndrome accounting for the bone-tiredness so frequently experienced.

Deficiency

The major symptom of a CoQ10 deficiency is fatigue. I use this nutrient extensively in the clinic to treat chronic fatigue syndrome. Other indications that our CoQ10 may be low are cardiovascular problems, especially electrical arrhythmia and cardiac-muscular dysfunction.

Antagonists

Cholesterol-lowering drugs (collectively known as statin drugs) are to date the only known source of opposition (see following page).

Sources

CoQ10 is found in oily fish, organ meats and whole grains.

Recommended therapeutic dose

To achieve a significant increase in energy, we need at least 60 mg per day. Ideally 30 mg three to four times per day would achieve a good clinical result. Dosages used in heart disease are between 50 and 600 mg daily, although in the normal ageing heart 100 mg per day is effective.

Coenzyme Q10 and cholesterol-lowering drugs

Cholesterol-lowering drugs, collectively known as the statin drugs, lower cholesterol by blocking an enzyme known by the peculiar alphabetic conglomeration of HMG CoA reductase. Unfortunately, this also reduces the body's own production of CoQ10, which, of course, can lead to fatigue.

So it is especially important for patients taking statin drugs to also take CoQ10. It has been proven indispensable to cardiac function, and congestive cardiac failure is viewed as a principal symptom of CoQ10 deficiency. A recent study has shown that even brief exposure to statin drugs (two weeks) can cause a marked decrease in blood CoQ10 concentration. It has been speculated that the inhibition of CoQ10 synthesis may explain the common side effects of the statin drugs; such as exercise intolerance, muscle fatigue and the occasional positive finding of haemoglobin in the urine. An effective dose to offset the CoQ10-lowering effects of the statin drugs would be 100 mg daily.

CHAPTER EIGHT

Mental clarity
and agility

Nutrition for maximum mental clarity

A healthy diet is crucial in achieving clarity of thought and a memory in tip-top condition. Although the brain represents only 6 per cent of body weight, it consumes between a quarter to a third of the body's oxygen and blood sugar. A most metabolically active body part! Sugar is converted into energy in the mitochondria (energy power house of the cell), and then transported to the brain where it is turned into essential neurotransmitters. As Dr George Watson in his classic tome *Nutrition and Your Mind* so succinctly explains, 'What one eats, digests and assimilates, provides the energy-producing nutrients that the bloodstream carries to the brain. What you eat determines your state of mind and who you are.'

Let's look at key nutrients used to enhance mental alertness and banish brain fatigue and fogginess. Bear in mind, however, that being well hydrated, exercising regularly and maintaining a well-balanced diet is a good starting point to maximise mental perception and potential.

Phenylalanine
Description
This is an amino acid used in the production of two key neurotransmitters that promote alertness: dopamine and noradrenalin. It can elevate mood, improve memory and learning, decrease pain and suppress appetite. Phenylalanine is an essential amino acid; it cannot be produced by our liver and must be obtained through the diet.

Phenylalanine is required for brain and nerve function. It is also the precursor for the production of tyrosine, another amino acid that affects brain function. Tyrosine supplementation has been shown to have positive effects on physical performance and cognitive function, especially during periods of stress. Phenylalanine assists in the production of thyroid and adrenal hormones, which are essential in helping us to deal with stress. Low adrenal hormones can be likened to having no booster rockets when you need to get out of trouble, or having no ability to bounce back. It's the most common cause of burnout.

Recommended therapeutic dose

The RTD is 500 mg per day. Taken on an empty stomach with fruit juice will ensure it crosses the blood–brain barrier.

Caution: Avoid in cases of Phenylketonuria – a rare metabolic disorder in which phenylalanine cannot be converted to tyrosine, causing nerve function problems. Phenylalanine should also not be taken by pregnant women, or people who have pre-existing pigmented melanoma. Caution also in cases of high blood pressure and diabetes.

Glutamine

Description

Glutamine is commonly known as brain fuel and is used to increase mental alertness and concentration span. Glutamic acid, which is converted to glutamine, is the only amino acid metabolised in the brain, where it is found in high concentrations. Glutamine lowers levels of ammonia in brain tissue, which improves brain function and memory.

Glutamine is also found in muscle tissue and when the body runs low in glutamine it will strip down and use muscle tissue to obtain more of it. As a matter of course, I put my triathlete clients on a glutamine regime prior to an intense period of training. The last thing any athlete wants is to break down muscle tissue to obtain more of it! Glutamine is also required for an efficient immune system, and poor immunity in hard-training sports people is often due to low reserves of glutamine.

Glutamine is used to treat fatigue, senility, Parkinsonism, a range of developmental disabilities and alcoholism. It decreases sugar and alcohol cravings. Glutamine combines with vitamin B6 and manganese to form the precursor to the neurotransmitter GABA (gamma-amino butyric acid), which has a relaxing effect on the central nervous system and is used to treat anxiety.

Glutamine provides fuel for intestinal cells and is used extensively in the repair of leaky-gut syndrome, and therefore may help to improve the absorption of nutrients.

Recommended therapeutic dose

The RTD is 500–1000 mg per day taken on an empty stomach. (I can personally vouch for this one. I used it for short bursts when I was studying and noticed a significant improvement in memory retention and recall.)

Caution: Avoid in cases of kidney and liver disease, and Reye's syndrome.

Aspartic acid
Description

Aspartic acid is a major element in the energy cycle of the body and it is a useful supplement to increase resistance to fatigue and improve stamina. It provides energy by being converted to glucose, the simplest and most easy-to-use energy source of the body. Low levels of aspartic acid results in lowered cellular energy. This amino acid, found in high levels in the brain, stimulates nerve cells, relieves mental fatigue, increases mental perception, and has a beneficial effect on brain and neural disorders. It also combines with other amino acids to form molecules that absorb and remove toxins from the bloodstream. By removing ammonia and other muscle waste products from the system it naturally increases resistance to fatigue.

As well as being found in its amino acid form of L-aspartic acid, it is also available in magnesium, potassium, calcium and zinc salts. In combination with magnesium, as magnesium aspartate, it plays an important role in the production of energy by transporting magnesium into the cells. It is used extensively in the treatment of chronic fatigue syndrome and, in a number of clinical studies, has dramatically improved energy levels within six weeks of constant use.

Sources
Aspartic acid is found in most protein foods. In its aspar-agines form, it is found in abundance in plants, especially sprouted seeds, such as sesame, pumpkin, sunflower and alfalfa.

Recommended therapeutic dose
The RTD is 1000 mg two times per day.

Choline
Description
Choline is often referred to as the 'memory' vitamin as without choline brain function and memory are impaired. Indeed, it is one of the few vitamins able to cross the blood–brain barrier and is directly involved in chemical reactions in the brain. Choline is part of the neurotransmitter, acetylcholine, which helps the electrical transmission of brain impulses from nerves to muscles and organs.

Choline is also one of the lipotropic B-group vitamins – that is, it helps the body to emulsify fats and cholesterol. So, not only does choline assist in overcoming mental fatigue through its impact on the nervous system, it also helps in weight control through the breakdown of fats – a wondrous vitamin indeed!

The 'brain fog' experienced in CFS can be treated by increasing the levels of choline. Choline has also produced some encouraging results in the treatment of Alzheimer's disease; these include improvement in behaviour and memory, and better upper-limb coordination. Several of my clients have been using high doses of choline to improve memory function and clear-headedness with great results.

Sources

Phosphatidyl choline is a basic component of soy lecithin. Other sources include egg yolk, brewer's yeast, wheat-germ, fish, leafy greens and organ meats. If large amounts of lecithin are taken, more calcium is required to balance the phosphorus found in lecithin.

Recommended therapeutic dose

The RTD is 500–1000 mg, and it is best taken with the other B-group vitamins.

HERBS AND MENTAL AGILITY

Before we officially look at herbal medicine and its role in the treatment of fatigue, let's take a sneak preview at two herbs specific to mental acuity: *Ginkgo biloba* and *Bacopa monnieri*.

We now know that the amino acids phenylalanine,

glutamine and aspartic acid, plus the B-group vitamin choline, can help us achieve maximum efficiency from each of our brain cells; but we also have the wonderful world of herbs to assist us in this, if you will pardon the pun, grey matter.

Bacopa (*Bacopa monnieri*)

This gorgeous herb is also known by its Sanskrit name of *brahmi*, although its common English name is water hyssop.

Bacopa, in recent years, has received a great deal of interest for its reputation as a brain and nerve tonic. Traditionally we have used bacopa for improving memory, concentration and learning, especially where stress is present. Bacopa has also been used to assist in the intellectual development of children; to repair neuronal deficit due to injury or stroke; to treat Alzheimer's disease; and it is valuable in the treatment of nervous exhaustion and conditions where anxiety may play a part, such as irritable bowel syndrome.

Clinical trials with this herb have been extremely encouraging. In a trial lasting a month involving thirty-five patients with anxiety neurosis, bacopa significantly reduced anxiety and improved mental performance. This increased mental performance was accompanied by a reduction in mental fatigue, a general feeling of well-being, improved sleep and appetite. Likewise, bacopa significantly improved IQ scores of ten- to thirteen-year-old children, with average intelligence, over a treatment period of nine months.

A memory and anxiety study undertaken in 2002, involving seventy-six adults aged between forty and sixty-five, showed that bacopa had a significant effect on the retention of new information. Follow-up tests suggested a decreased rate of forgetting the newly acquired information. These, and other clinical results, are very encouraging; mental fatigue and anxiety have a detrimental effect on memory, and bacopa has proved beneficial in treating the underlying cause as well as the symptoms.

In order to benefit from the brain-tonic effects of this herb, a treatment time of at least six weeks, and preferably twelve weeks, is necessary. A steady improvement in memory recall and learning should be discernible by the eight-week mark.

Ginkgo (*Ginkgo biloba*)

I love this tree. It is one of the oldest living plant species; fossils have been dated as far back as 250 million years ago. Charles Darwin called it the 'living fossil', and it is so resilient that it was the first tree to reappear in Hiroshima after the bombing. The leaves of the ginkgo tree have been used in China for many centuries to treat age-related illness. In France and Germany, ginkgo extract is one of the major prescriptive medicines, and is rebatable on the national-health schemes of these countries. Ginkgo tends to concentrate in brain tissue, and it is interesting to note that the leaf of the ginkgo tree has a startling resemblance to a cross-section of the cerebellum, the second-largest part of the human brain. (This is referred to as the Doctrine of Signatures in herbal medicine: a plant resembles the body part it affects or heals. Another example would be *dong quai*: the root resembles the uterus and is used to treat female reproductive problems.)

Ginkgo works in different ways to bacopa, but similarly improves memory and banishes mental fatigue. Being a circulatory stimulant, ginkgo improves blood supply to the brain and, therefore, enhances oxygen supply to the nervous tissue. Extracts of gingko are used to treat poor brain oxygenation, which could manifest as one or all of the following: difficulty with concentration and memory, absentmindedness, confusion, anxiety and headache; these days it is being used in Western medicine to treat Alzheimer's disease. It is also a potent anti-oxidant, inhibits platelet aggregation (stops cells sticking together) and has been used with some success in treating dementia due to nerve cell degeneration, by decreasing oxidative damage. Indeed, the flavonoids in ginkgo are ten times more potent free-radical scavengers than those in blueberries or citrus peel. In elderly patients it has been shown to reduce symptoms of vertigo, tinnitus, memory loss and headache. Ginkgo is excellent for older people living in colder climates.

Ginkgo has been shown to increase glucose absorption in some areas of the brain and to help nerve cells in the forebrain absorb the nutrient choline from the blood. And, as we have just discussed, choline also improves brain function and memory. Recent studies have demonstrated that ginkgo slows the deterioration of nerve cell receptors, which increases the serotonin uptake and raises the production of noradrenalin, one of our adrenal hormones.

Psychological testing of people using a herbal extract of ginkgo at the Brain Sciences Institute (BSI; Swinburne University of Technology, Melbourne, Victoria), indicates that significant improvements in working memory, and in the speed of the brain's information processing can be achieved with this herb.

The 2002 trial involved fifty-five participants aged between eighteen and forty. They were tested on a battery of psychological tasks assessing intelligence, concentration, attention, memory, problem solving, speed of visual information processing and social intelligence before and after consuming either a ginkgo extract or a placebo.

The results showed that participants with average IQs who took ginkgo improved attention and problem-solving capacity significantly more than those with higher IQs. Indeed, the scores of those with lower IQs in tests of attention increased to almost the same level as the performance of the higher IQ group.

These results suggest that in healthy people, ginkgo administered for thirty days can significantly boost a range of intellectual characteristics.

Caution: Avoid ginkgo when taking aspirin, Warfarin and Haloperidol. Discontinue taking ginkgo seven days prior to surgery.

CHAPTER NINE

Herbal medicine

Plants have been used as medicines since antiquity, and the herbal kingdom has been particularly generous in providing us with an enormous array of choices in the treatment of fatigue. Herbs are a safe, natural, effective means of both helping to increase energy and in treating the underlying cause of fatigue. The herbs we prescribe are classified as 'nervine relaxants', 'nervine tonics' and the 'adaptogenic' herbs. Let's look at a couple of examples from each category to provide an insight into how and when they are used.

Nervine relaxants

When stress and tension are the major factors in causing fatigue – either through the indirect impact they have on our nutrient status and adrenal function or, more directly, their effect on our sleeping patterns – the relaxant herbs are appropriate to use.

A representative list of herbs used in the clinic would include: passionflower (*Passiflora incarnata*), lime flowers (*Tilia europa*), chamomile (*Matricaria recutita*), St John's wort (*Hypericum perforatum*), skullcap (*Scutellaria laterifolia*) and valerian (*Valeriana officinalis*). Let's consider in more detail the relaxant herbs skullcap and passionflower.

Skullcap (*Scutellaria laterifolia*)

Skullcap has a relaxing and gentle sedative effect on the nervous system. It relaxes nervous tension while, at the same time, renewing and revitalising the central nervous system. It can be used in all exhaustion-related and depressive conditions, and is also effective in treating panic and anxiety attacks, particularly when there is an element of hysteria.

I usually prescribe skullcap in conditions marked by nervous tension, stress and/or exhaustion. It is extremely beneficial in cases of poor concentration due to fatigue and anxiety, and where there is poor digestion and dyspepsia as a result of nervous tension.

Passionflower (*Passiflora incarnata*)

Passionflower is a traditional folk remedy for anxiety. It has performed magnificently in recent clinical trials that compare it with the drug Oxazepam, in the treatment of generalised anxiety disorder. The study showed that both our herbal friend and the drug were effective in the treatment of anxiety. Oxazepam provided faster results, however, the subjects taking the drug encountered more problems relating to impaired job performance.

Passionflower's antispasmodic effect makes it the ideal remedy for stress-related abdominal pain or spasm. Its natural sedative qualities are especially valuable in the treatment of anxiety; for instance, calming that racing heart so often associated with nervousness, as well as irritability and exhaustion due to broken sleep. It has been shown to improve the quality of sleep.

Caution: Not to be taken during pregnancy. Be careful if taken with benzodiazepines as the sedative effects of the drug may be increased.

NERVINE TONICS

The herbs in this category represent the most important contribution herbal medicine can make in strengthening and feeding the nervous system. Nervine tonics revitalise. The herbs I normally prescribe are oats (*Avena sativa*), damiana (*Turnera aphrodisiaca*) and vervain (*Verbena officinalis*), and we will focus on oats and damiana.

Oat seed (*Avena sativa*)

Oat is one of the best remedies to nourish nervous tissue and the nervous system. It is used to treat cases of nervous exhaustion and debility, especially when associated with depression. Its ability to 'feed' the nervous system makes it a wonderful herb to use in situations where there has been considerable stress over a long period of time.

From a naturopathic point of view, not only is oat a nervine tonic but it is also classified as a demulcent, having a soothing effect on mucous membranes, thereby reducing symptoms of gut-wall irritation; it also has the ability to heal wounds. The high levels of the mineral silica found in the oat plant means that it may also be used, both internally and externally, as a remedy for skin conditions (silica is present in bone, blood vessels and hair).

Oat can either be taken directly in the form of tinctures or teas, or combined in a herbal mixture with other relaxant remedies. Or, of course, it can simply be eaten in the form of old-fashioned porridge. And all good Scotsmen and women can vouch for the power of the oat! (See APPENDIX ELEVEN The power of the oat! for a nutritional analysis of oats and some inspiring oat recipes.)

Oat, in the tincture form, is used extensively in the clinic. I regularly incorporate it in herbal mixtures to treat the nervous system, irritable bowel (or any gut discomfort with an anxiety component) and some skin conditions. People with a gluten sensitivity can tolerate the tincture (gluten is found in wheat, oats, barley and rye).

Damiana (*Turnera aphrodisiaca*)

As you can tell from the second part of this delightful plant's Latin name, it has an ancient reputation as an aphrodisiac. While there is no scientific proof to support this reputation (the alkaloids of this plant *may* have a testosterone-like action), it is certainly not an unappealing benefit!

However, damiana's real strength lies in its ability to bolster the nervous system. It is an excellent nerve tonic and anti-depressant and ideal to use in cases of long-term anxiety and depression, chronic debilitation of the central nervous system and for sexual inadequacies that have a strong emotional element. Damiana is said to provide a mild euphoria and to improve stamina. Simon Mills, a world-renowned authority on herbalism and member of the British Herbal Medicine Association, so articulately describes damiana when he says, '. . . it often fills a desirable place in a prescription for those simply too sad.'

ADAPTOGENS

The adaptogenic group of herbs is one of the most appropriate in the treatment of fatigue, both preventively and symptomatically. An adaptogen is a substance that increases an organism's resistance to physical, chemical and biological stressors. This term and definition was introduced by Nikolai Lazarev, a Russian pharmacologist, in 1947. Since then, the study of adaptogens has attracted an enormous amount of attention, indeed, it has become a field of biomedical research in its own right. In China and India adaptogens form the very basis of their preventative approach to health and wellbeing.

By strengthening the adrenal gland (and possibly the pituitary gland) the adaptogenic herbs enable the body to cope with the adverse effects of long-term stress. They help us avoid reaching a point of collapse – also referred to as 'adrenal exhaustion'. A great number of adaptogens also stimulate the immune system, and have a discernable influence on increasing a sense of wellbeing.

Adaptogens, similar to the old-fashioned tonics, are often prescribed at times in our lives when stress is high or during particularly difficult periods of change. This category of herbs includes panax ginseng, Siberian ginseng, withania, astragalus, schisandra, bacopa and liquorice root – no, not the commercial type! My favourite and most widely used adaptogenic herb in the clinic is *Eleutherococcus senticosus*; that is, Siberian ginseng.

Siberian Ginseng (*Eleutherococcus senticosus*)

Siberian ginseng is essentially a restorative herb. It increases energy and resistance in those who are debilitated or stressed, and assists us to withstand adverse physical conditions.

Clinical trials using Siberian ginseng on healthy individuals have shown increased performance and stamina. Mental and physical output is increased; for example, proofreaders are quicker and make fewer errors and labourers are more productive. It has been widely used by Russian athletes for its ability to increase concentration and improve performance. When given to cancer patients it minimised the side-effects from radiation, chemotherapy and surgery, and improved healing and wellbeing.

Combined with withania, bacopa and rosemary, Siberian ginseng has quite measurable beneficial effects on mental performance and memory, while improving stamina and alleviating the effects of nervous exhaustion on mental function. It is gently calming and also elevates mood by treating any depression associated with fatigue.

Caution: Take with care in the presence of hypertension; avoid in pregnancy and lactation, and in combination with anticoagulants, such as Warfarin; and discontinue seven days prior to surgery.

Withania (*Withania somnifera*)

Withania, also known as Indian ginseng, winter cherry or *ashwagandha*, is a superb adaptogenic tonic. It has a mild sedative effect and is most suitable in cases of nervous exhaustion, debility associated with chronic stress, anxiety and depression. It is also rich in iron. Interestingly, the name *ashwagandha* literally means 'smell of a horse'; it is believed that the name refers to the herb traditionally being used to build a person's strength and resilience to equal that of a horse!

Withania is used extensively in Ayurvedic medicine (an ancient Indian medicine that has its roots in a 2000-year-old tradition) and is categorised as a 'vasagna'; that is, it promotes physical and mental health, protects against disease and adverse environmental factors, and arrests the ageing process. What more could a herbalist hope for! A study investigating the anti-depressant and anti-anxiety actions of withania showed it to have an anti-depressant effect in situations marked by despair and feelings of helplessness. Withania has also been shown to reduce hyperglycaemia, glucose intolerance, gastric ulceration, male sexual dysfunction and immune suppression – all factors that may be induced by chronic stress.

Withania is an ideal tonic for the physically active or the elderly, as well as being one of the key herbs used to treat chronic fatigue syndrome.

Note: A clinical trial investigating the effects of one of the individual constituents of withania (sitoindosides) found that oral administration of withania protected rats against stress-induced stomach ulcers.

Gota kola (*Centella asiatica*)

Many will be familiar with the Sanskrit term *brahmi*: it refers to a combination of Ayurvedic herbs, available in tablet form from health food shops, designed to improve memory. Gota kola is one of these herbs. It is a brilliant adaptogenic herb, especially suitable for use in cases of mental fatigue and anxiety. It is a gentle cerebral stimulant – and there will always be times in our lives when we need to gently nudge the grey matter! According to Ayurvedic tradition it revitalises nerves and brain cells, increases mental performance, improves memory, strengthens the adrenals and decreases senility and ageing. This wonderful herb is often combined with ginkgo – also known for its positive effect on memory, due to its ability to increase blood supply to the brain. Indeed, when combined with ginkgo and bacopa it has a powerful effect on improving memory and concentration.

I frequently prescribe gota kola in situations where there is a foreseen period of prolonged stress and where mental agility is paramount; for example, public performances and deadlines for major projects – especially publishers' deadlines! It is lovely to learn that this herb is found in the Himalayas where it is used by yogis to assist meditation.

Veronica had recently had the rather frightening experience of feeling so dizzy that she needed to concentrate very carefully on each step in order to make her way slowly back home after an afternoon out shopping. She told me she was uncharacteristically snappy, easily frazzled and 'on edge'; and that she had become increasingly dependent on sleeping tablets following her marriage break-up five years ago.

Veronica is a very active fifty-year-old woman, walking and samba dancing regularly, as well as teaching English to final-year high school students. Her diet is quite good, with just a few too many coffees and a variable water intake. Despite spending long periods in confined spaces with young adults five days a week, she rarely comes down with a cold or the flu. However, at the end of the mid-semester term she had several episodes of these dizzy spells, was tired and anxious, and was having increasing difficulty in sleeping. Veronica's iris analysis revealed a strong constitution, a slightly acidic tendency and fairly chronic physiological stress (she had well-entrenched 'nerve arcs', that is circular grooves in the outer region of her iris). Blood tests revealed good levels of iron, B12 and folate; and her blood pressure was 120/80. So, we could rule out anaemia or low-blood pressure contributing to her dizziness and fatigue.

Veronica was, in fact, on the edge of adrenal exhaustion. Fortunately, her strong constitution, good diet and regular exercise had prevented a more rapid deterioration. I prescribed a herbal mixture that included withania, Siberian ginseng, bacopa and vervain; this would restore and support the adrenals, as well as have a calming and relaxing effect on the nervous system. I advised Veronica to take a good-quality vitamin-B-plus-C formula to provide the base nutrients for adrenal function. We agreed that she would stop using the sleeping tablets (she was in the habit of using half a tablet at least four times per week, 'just in case I can't get to sleep'), and I gave her a herbal sedative formula to use each night over the next few weeks while we re-adjusted and restored her normal sleeping patterns. Her dose was 7 ml of the sleep mixture one hour before bed and then a further 7 ml at bedtime. If she woke up during the night she could take a further measured dose. (No estimating, always use a measuring cup to ensure the prescribed dose is taken when using herbal medicine. A teaspoon is *not* 7 ml.) This mixture would ensure a restful night's sleep without morning grogginess or fear of addiction. All coffee and tea after two o'clock in the afternoon was banned – not good for the adrenals or a sound night's sleep.

Fortunately, at the time of our first consultation Veronica was on holiday, so she had a few weeks to implement and benefit from her herbal treatment without the stressors of the normal weekly rush. Within two weeks Veronica was feeling less anxious and irritable, and within four weeks she was sleeping well without sleeping tablets or herbs. At the eight-week mark Veronica was feeling 'fantastic . . . like my old self again', full of energy and enthusiasm in the mornings, and no signs of dizziness or edginess. We discontinued the herbs after twelve weeks. Veronica now takes a strong multi-vitamin daily, is careful to drink at least 2 litres of water a day, and takes time out from that exhausting mental chatter by beginning each day with yoga, in the privacy of her lounge room. The last time I saw Veronica she was bursting with vitality, enthusiastic about her work, waking up feeling refreshed and looking fantastic.

ADRENAL GLAND TONIC

An example of a herbal mixture I may put together at the clinic to treat a client suffering from debilitating fatigue with a stress component would look something like this:

Siberian ginseng	*35 ml*
Withania	*35 ml*
Oats	*20 ml*
*Liquorice root	*15 ml*

This herbal mixture would be taken three times per day at a dose of 5 ml over a period of three to six months.

Rosemary, bacopa or ginkgo could be added or substituted to enhance mental performance. If there was irritability and tension, especially in conditions that have persisted long enough to result in depressive fatigue, then I would add St John's wort. St John's wort has been found to have the same efficacy as some anti-depressant drugs affecting neurotransmitter concentrations in the brain.

Do not self-administer St John's wort as there are a number of adverse interactions with this herb and some pharmaceuticals, such as oral contraceptives, anti-depressants, Warfarin, protease inhibitors, some hypoglycaemic and cholesterol medications, and reverse transcriptase inhibitors. The main consequence is a possible decreased efficacy of these medications. If unsure seek advice from your naturopath or herbalist.

Note: Liquorice root has a direct effect on adrenal production. It encourages the production of cortisol by the adrenal cortex. Cortisol ensures there is an adequate fuel supply to the cell when the body is under stress. Liquorice has a very long history in herbal medicine, being used by Western, Chinese, Kanpo and Ayurvedic herbalists. Chinese herbalists use it in mixtures to help increase the absorption and effect of the other herbs.

A herbalist would find it difficult to run an efficient dispensary without this herb. I probably use more liquorice root in my practice than any other herb. And, it has a bonus – it is actually very pleasant tasting, and often helps to make a rather unpalatable herbal mixture far more appealing: 'Just a spoonful of liquorice helps the herbal mixture go down!'

The beauty of herbal medicine is that it can be tailored to suit each individual and changed as symptoms improve or other health issues come up. People really do become attached to their herbs and genuinely miss them when treatment has finished. It's true!

CHAPTER TEN

THE STRESS FACTOR

WHAT IS STRESS?

Stress is the individual physiological and emotional response by our body to any demand made on it. It is a non-specific response to any stimuli that requires us to change or adapt in some way; a condition caused by a demand that exceeds our own unique coping abilities. And seeing that one of the great certainties of life is change, some degree of stress is pretty much unavoidable!

A stressor may be physical (such as heat, cold, a bleeding wound), chemical (pollutants, food additives) or emotional (relationships, work pressures). Our initial response to perceived stressors triggers the 'flight or fight' mechanism. The response – to stay and battle or flee from danger – is largely dependent on the adrenal glands: an intricate biochemical–hormonal process.

Stress itself is not a disease, but it is the way we choose, or have learned, to respond to stress that can be so detrimental to our health.

PHYSIOLOGICAL EFFECTS OF STRESS

Dr Hans Selye, the endocrinologist who in 1946 developed the stress concept and mapped its physiology, found that four organs are affected by stress: the adrenal glands become enlarged and bloodshot; the thymus and lymph glands (responsible for our immune response) atrophy, and the gastric mucosa become spotted with bleeding ulcers. It is hardly surprising, therefore, that stressful periods in our lives often result in sheer adrenal exhaustion, lowered immunity, digestive disorders and discomfort.

The stress response, via the stimulation of adrenal hormones, affects the metabolic rate and water balance. Adrenalin stimulates the heart, increasing blood pressure and heart rate; it constricts blood vessels, increasing the blood flow to the muscles and the brain and decreasing it to the digestive tract. Adrenalin also raises blood-sugar levels and stimulates the liver to release more glucose and cholesterol into the blood. Not an ideal physiological state to be in for a prolonged period of time; sadly, a great many people are, due to a sense of constant, unrelenting threats.

A feeling of vague unease seems to permeate the

everyday lives of a great many people, this is often a manifestation of a perceived lack of time and too many demands. More worrying is the finding that even people who are *not* aware of feeling stressed actually show physiological signs of stress. Swiss researchers, evaluating the stress response in nurses and physicians in a hospital environment who claimed to have no conscious perception of stress, found that salivary cortisol levels in the subjects (stress increases the secretion of cortisol by the adrenal glands) were more than 200 per cent above average.

Let's examine the physiological effects of stress a little more closely. It is truly amazing to discover the enormous impact our reaction to everyday stressors can have on our wellbeing. We are all very aware of the signs and symptoms of acute stress. Our heart rate increases, our breathing becomes rapid and shallow, our mouth becomes dry, our digestive function freezes and the blood supply to the skin and viscera (except the lungs) is withdrawn. If the stressful situation is quickly resolved our body soon returns to normal. If, however, the stress is prolonged – such as a stressful job, financial hardship, irresolvable relationship issues, or never-ending and demanding work deadlines – our body remains in this alert physiological state, which uses up all of our nutritional and energy resources. Chronic stress results in the serious condition of nutritional deficiency and burnout; a total shutdown of the adrenal glands occurs and the end result is exhaustion.

How much stress can we handle?

Hans Selye saw the body's capacity to handle stress as finite and much more important than the actual stress itself. In other words, we have an individual tolerance level, or a set supply of energy for life, and once used up, it is gone forever. So the way we respond to stress has crucial implications for our precious energy reserves and long-term wellbeing.

Selye described our ability to withstand chronic stress as unsustainable, like deep deposits of oil – once burned up, gone forever. Consequently, a high-stress lifestyle means our supply is spent rapidly and we age faster. Prolonged stress puts an enormous load on many organs; especially the heart, adrenal glands, blood vessels and the immune system. As a result, we become candidates for early coronary heart disease, strokes, ulcers, bowel disease, auto-immune diseases and chronic fatigue; we even become more accident prone. Our internalised response to stress thus becomes physiologically destructive. It has been estimated that 90 per cent of disease is directly caused by, or complicated by, stress. I feel quite comfortable in saying that, from my own clinical observation, most people's poor health, particularly fatigue, is directly attributable to stress and diet.

Seyle recognised a common pattern in the stress response and called it the General Adaptation Syndrome. He identified three phases of stress – the alarm, resistance and exhaustion phases. The *first phase*: the initial encounter with stress, which could be physical as well as mental, stimulates the release of stress hormones, such as adrenalin, in order to rise to the challenge. If the stress continues, however, there will be a *second phase*: one of resistance, when the body acclimatises to the stress. This stage involves considerable expenditure of energy, increasing pressure on the adrenal gland (particularly the adrenal cortex that secretes cortisol) to meet emotional crises, fight infection or perform strenuous tasks. Prolonged stress will eventually lead to the *third phase* in the General Adaptation Syndrome: exhaustion, which marks the onset of many diseases. The stress response that was originally physiologically stimulating becomes irreversibly debilitating and major systemic deterioration sets in. There will be total adrenal shutdown and other organs, such as the heart and the immune system, may also collapse. Hence we have a finite vital capacity to deal with unrelenting stress.

Given the fact that many people feel they are under

constant pressure – whether this is in the work environment meeting a steady stream of deadlines; or in the home, transporting children, organising meals, overseeing homework – it is not surprising that many of us are genuinely physiologically, really and truly tired.

Naturopaths often refer to the 'vital force'. It can best be described as our innate constitutional capacity: our physical, mental, emotional and spiritual energy. Most naturopathic consultations involve an iris analysis – an examination of the iris using a magnifying glass with a light. One of the first areas we look at is the iris structure; that is, the way the fibres radiate from the pupil, like spokes of a wheel. This pattern indicates our constitution or inherited resilience: the denser the fibres the stronger the constitution and the greater our ability to bounce back. How we age can also be used to measure our vital force: those who stay fit and healthy in old age are the most successful in preserving their adrenal-based strength. We need to understand the concept of 'vital force' in order to recognise that fatigue is often the result of the interaction between stress and potential disease, and the body's powers of self-recuperation.

 It was obvious when Elizabeth came to the clinic that she had recently had a bad accident. She had two surgical sticking plasters taped across the bridge of her nose, two black eyes and multiple scratches over her forehead. Her reasons for coming to see me, however, had nothing to do with her recent injuries, rather she had made the appointment to help her insomnia. I discovered during the consultation that she had recently lost her appetite, was having increasingly frequent attacks of nervous asthma and tachycardia (rapid heart beat) and, in her own words, was on the 'edge of going under'. She was feeling emotionally overwhelmed and physically exhausted.

Elizabeth is in her mid-fifties; active, she walks daily and plays tennis twice-weekly, has a busy social life and a very close extended family. In recent years Elizabeth has been increasingly called upon by members of her grown-up family for emotional support and practical help; including babysitting, shopping, financial assistance, as well as arranging frequent family social events.

Her facial injuries were a result of walking through French doors at home. At the time, her husband had just had exploratory surgery and they were waiting for the results, plus her daughter was in hospital having her tonsils removed, leaving Elizabeth with two very young grandchildren to look after. She admitted that she had probably not eaten very much on the day of the accident and had almost certainly been dehydrated. Remember that stressed people are far more accident prone.

Elizabeth's insomnia, or more accurately her maintenance insomnia (she can get to sleep but wakes up throughout the night), began about six years ago, shortly after her mother passed away, but had recently become much worse. She was waking up almost hourly from two o'clock in the morning onwards.

I immediately prescribed a vitamin B complex twice daily, one with breakfast and one with lunch; and one calcium tablet before dinner and two at bedtime. These very basic adjustments would soothe the nervous system, help reduce anxiety and assist with sleep. I made up a herbal sleep formula consisting of: passionflower, valerian, hops and California poppy, all gentle nervous system relaxants with a strong sedative component; 7 ml to be taken one hour before bed, 7 ml at bedtime and a further dose if she woke up during the night. I also put Elizabeth on an adrenal nutritional formula comprising: vitamin B5 (an essential nutrient for cortisol formation, the hormone secreted by the adrenal gland that regulates stress), vitamin B6, vitamin C and magnesium. These nutrients in particular can be rapidly depleted during periods of stress.

Due to the rather acute nature of Elizabeth's situation, I made up a homeopathic Bach flower formula (see CHAPTER FOURTEEN) to address her feeling of being overwhelmed with responsibility, her physical exhaustion and her fearfulness for the health of her family. She was to take four drops on the tongue four times per day. I also strongly recommended that Elizabeth start on a good-quality vitamin E capsule, and to apply the oil locally to her wounds to prevent any facial scarring.

Elizabeth's diet was generally very well balanced, so the only adjustments I needed to make were to totally exclude caffeine and encourage an increased consumption of lovely, grounding high-potassium root vegetables. And NO skipping meals! Elizabeth needed to eat three meals per day, with a fruit or yoghurt snack mid-morning and mid-afternoon. It was important to keep her blood-sugar levels stable, as hypoglycaemia can provoke palpitations and light-headedness. She also promised to measure her water consumption to make sure she was drinking 2 litres per day. (I often find with clients who are on the go all day, without a regular daily routine, that water intake is inadequate. It is easy to 'forget' to drink when you are rushing around, in and out of the car all day long. My suggestion is to place two large bottles of water in the car, and with constant swigging, both bottles should be empty by the end of the day.)

Two weeks later, when Elizabeth returned for a follow-up consultation, she certainly looked a lot better. The facial swelling had subsided and she was healing well. Happily her sleep had also improved, and she was now generally sleeping right through with just the occasional night of interrupted sleep. I advised her to continue with the sleep mixture for a further week just to be sure we had well and truly broken her poor sleeping habit, and then to use the herbs only if she woke up during the night. The episodes of tachycardia had totally disappeared and the asthma had substantially subsided, but was still occurring every couple of days. I therefore prescribed a high-dose magnesium supplement to help further relax the nervous system and, in particular, the bronchials. Elizabeth continued for another four weeks on the adrenal support formula and maintained the twice-a-day B complex as part of her 'constitutional' remedy. Once the homeopathic formula was finished it could be discontinued.

One month later, Elizabeth was sleeping well without the herbs, her normally strong appetite had returned, the asthma was largely under control and she was much more relaxed. I strongly recommended she start meditation classes so that future episodes of stress would not have the same impact.

STRESS MANAGEMENT

Although everyone responds to stress differently, Elizabeth's regimen was pretty typical of how to treat it. Increasing the intake of B-group vitamins, together with vitamin C and magnesium, is crucial as these nutrients are all swiftly used up during periods of stress. Herbs such as verbena, lime flowers, chamomile and lemon balm have a wonderfully relaxing action on the nervous system and can help soothe frayed nerves. Strong sedative herbs, such as passionflower, valerian, California poppy and hops, may be necessary for short periods in our lives when stress disturbs our sleeping patterns.

For periods of prolonged stress the adaptogen group of herbs has no rival! These herbs, which include Siberian ginseng, panax ginseng and withania, have a stabilising impact on the body and help us to adapt to new situations and changed environments. Their protective and restorative characteristics increase our resistance to stress and, importantly, are gentle and safe to use. A herbal mixture can be tailored to specifically address the way stress manifests itself in you (see CHAPTER NINE Herbal medicine).

Other important stress management techniques include meditation, or similar relaxation practices, and exercise. Many studies support the mood-enhancing effect of exercise on the mind (think endorphins and enkephalins), and intense aerobic work-outs are now used to treat depression and anxiety (see CHAPTER ELEVEN Meditation to clear the mind, and CHAPTER THIRTEEN Exercise away fatigue). Breathing exercises are especially useful to control rapid, shallow breathing, which is a common symptom of anxiety; yoga or Pilates would be a superb way to learn and perfect your breathing techniques. However, exercise needs to be regular – that is *daily* – and our relaxation techniques have to be an integral part of our daily routine. Daily preventive measures, effortlessly incorporated into our lifestyles, are our insurance against the detrimental effects of our learned, but seldom questioned, response to stress.

In periods of stress, as well as following the healthy diet advice in CHAPTER THREE we need to avoid all stimulants – this includes caffeine, sugar and cigarettes. (Yes, tobacco is a stimulant and has a strong influence on the nervous system; there is NO situation where smoking is harmless.) It is particularly important to reduce the high-GI range of carbohydrates in the diet, thereby maintaining stable blood-sugar levels at all times (see APPENDIX ONE Glycaemic index).

Lastly, hands-on therapies such as massage, shiatsu and reflexology are also some calming considerations to help soothe an 'inflamed' nervous system and restore a sense of equilibrium. Spending an hour of our time being cared for by another using the tactile therapies is a safe and truly delightful way to address stress management.

CHAPTER ELEVEN

Meditation to clear the mind

Marrying the mind and body

Although certain vitamins and minerals, herbs and amino acids provide the raw materials for achieving mental clarity, clearness of thought and, indeed, action is also dependent on a calm, balanced energy. A sound nervous system ensures precise decision making as well as a fluid mind–body connection. Knocking things over and dropping things are indicators that our perception and movement are not well integrated. Anxiety produces an agitated and clouded mind.

Stilling the mind

How do we still the mind sufficiently to achieve clearness of mind and even breakthrough thinking? Strangely enough, the first step is to stop thinking! We need to stop the incessant mental chatter that prevents us from relaxing fully and causes us to toss and turn at night and lose precious sleep. Clarity arises from a clean slate. We all know that stilling the mind is, at first, no easy task but it does, thank goodness, get easier with practice. The key to quietening the mind, or to meditation, is not to tie yourself up in knots about it. You don't have to run around desperately trying to find the perfect technique, paying a fortune for secret mantras, or rigidly sitting in an uncomfortable lotus position willing the mind to stop. Relax. All you need to do is just put ten minutes aside each day to sit quietly and still the mind.

Meditation tips

An easy method is to sit comfortably, either in a chair or on a cushion on the floor, with your back reasonably straight, eyes either closed or lightly focused on the ground in front of you. Now, try to stop thinking. Every time a thought enters the mind, acknowledge it, gently push it to one side and return to clearing the mind. Thoughts will keep coming but don't try too hard to stop them or pay them much attention.

My initial attempts at meditation were frequently thwarted by an overconcern about the time. I found myself worrying that I was not sitting for long enough, or else I was sitting for too long (I had things to do and couldn't go too far over time, a classic example of someone who needs meditation!), so I put the oven timer on for ten minutes. This simple strategy had the positive result of stopping me thinking about the time issue while I was meditating. It is an unconventional approach, which would possibly be secretly sniggered at by more adept meditators, but it worked for me. After a few months I found I didn't need the oven timer dictating my session, as I seemed to naturally know when to stop.

The aim is simply to clear the mind and to quieten that constant mental chatter, which so often clouds our thoughts. As Daniel Reid, the author of several books including *The Complete Book of Chinese Health and Healing*, so eloquently puts it, 'It is the cerebral cortex that must be stilled and silenced in order to achieve mental clarity . . . for this is where the rambling train of nonstop thoughts hoots and toots noisily through the mind.'

Try to maintain a daily meditation routine, even if you feel that you are achieving very little; the benefits are great, despite our fears that we occasionally become distracted in the process. A soothing silence is actually a precious resource in a society where hyper-stimulation and noise is intrusive and just about unavoidable. Meditating for a few minutes at the end of the day is supremely valuable. Use a meditation method that works for you: watch your breath; use a mantra, creative visualisation or guided meditation; listen to a meditation CD; observe a candle or photograph of a deity. There are no right or wrong techniques, just the one which suits you. Practise until it becomes second nature and a pleasure to slip into.

CHAPTER TWELVE

SUCCESSFUL SLEEP

Lack of good-quality sleep zaps us of energy, so, if insomnia is becoming a pattern, try to identify and eliminate the causes. Establish routines that encourage healthy sleeping patterns and, if necessary, address any underlying nutritional inadequacies. Try to eliminate alcohol and caffeine completely for two weeks and compare the difference in your sleeping habits; exercise regularly, preferably in the morning; get out of bed at the same time every day; take a hot bath one to two hours before bed; and only go to bed when you are sleepy.

Sound sleeping habits are an important indicator of sound health. Falling asleep within ten minutes of lying down and sleeping peacefully for six to eight hours is important to our health. Sleep supports and rejuvenates our immune system and gives the nervous system time to 'catch up', and dispose of the waste products of metabolism.

Poor sleep results in fatigue and irritability; being deprived of sleep for a few days can lead to low immunity, disorientation and may eventually result in psychosis.

Stress and anxiety adversely affect sleep patterns. Cortisol, produced by our adrenal glands, rises dramatically with stress, triggering our body's 'fight or flight' response. Too much cortisol, as well as causing a weak malaise, can also interfere with sleep patterns, which ultimately produces a restless, non-restorative sleeping state. Waking up to a worn-out feeling is usually the result of adrenal exhaustion. (Remember our discussion in chapter seven of the importance of vitamins B5, B6 and C for supporting and feeding the adrenals.)

Most of my clients average six to seven hours of sleep on working days, and this seems to be the case amongst the general population. Compared to over a hundred years ago, when eight to nine hours was the norm, something has changed and not for the better. Even if falling asleep is not a problem, insufficient sleep appears to be a nationwide dilemma. Considering that one of the basic functions of sleep is to recuperate the body's metabolic functions, especially those affecting the brain, a country-wide fatigue is a real possibility. Brain glycogen stores that have been depleted during the waking hours are replenished during sleep. Long-term sleep deprivation may cause a cumulative sleep debt and seriously affect mental performance and judgement. Poor decision making and difficulty forming coherent, articulate sentences is a by-product of inadequate sleep.

Please avoid sleeping tablets. They *do not* cure insomnia, they can interfere with REM sleep, and continued use may lead to a disruption of the deeper stages of sleep. Research indicates that up to 50 per cent of people who take sleeping tablets on a regular basis find that their insomnia gets worse, and, as a consequence, it can result in dependency.

Insomnia – a resolution

There are two categories of habitual sleeplessness: 'Sleep onset insomnia' – difficulty falling asleep; and 'Maintenance insomnia' – frequent waking throughout the night. Of course, rarely does a health issue fit neatly into a single box, so there also exists a combination of the above two disorders.

Four steps to treat insomnia

1 | Identify and address possible causes of insomnia:

- anxiety
- pain
- depression

* caffeine
* alcohol
* tobacco (nicotine is a neurostimulant)
* environmental factors; e.g. barking dog, ventilation, bedroom too light
* food sensitivities
* breathing difficulties; e.g. sleep apnoea
* hypoglycaemia
* drugs; e.g. decongestants, appetite suppressants
* nutritional deficiencies.

2 | Establish regular routines to encourage restorative sleep:

* go to bed only when sleepy
* get out of bed at the same time every day
* do not nap during the day if this is not the norm for you
* exercise regularly, but avoid late-night work-outs
* take a hot bath one to two hours before bed.

3 | Nutritional and herbal therapy

There is a wide range of supplements available to us. The appropriate remedy will depend on your current dietary status and lifestyle demands.

Vitamin and mineral supplements:

* calcium and magnesium (1000 mg and 500 mg respectively) have a calming effect on the central nervous system and a relaxing effect on the muscular system. To be taken 45–60 minutes before bedtime;

* vitamin B complex with at least 50 mg of each of the B vitamins, taken in the morning, together with additional vitamin B5 (50 mg). Vitamin B5 is also helpful for those who grind their teeth at night;

* inositol (250–500 mg at bedtime) enhances REM sleep and decreases anxiety. Inositol is part of the vitamin B complex and, like choline, enhances brain cell nutrition.

Relaxant and sedative herbs:

* hops (*Humulus lupulus*)
* passionflower (*Passiflora incarnata*)
* skullcap (*Scutellaria laterifolia*)
* lemon balm (*Melissa officinalis*)
* chamomile (*Matricaria recutita*)
* California poppy (*Eschscholtzia californica*)
* valerian (*Valeriana officinalis*).*

The combination of a number of these herbs can help re-establish a regular sleep pattern, without the fear of addiction or grogginess in the morning. It is best to have a herbal mixture made up by your naturopath or herbalist to ensure the right dose and ratio of herbs is prescribed.

Note: Avoid using valerian in combination with barbiturates, and use with care with central nervous system depressant drugs as it may increase the drugs' effects.

Herbal teas

A cup of chamomile or lemon balm tea before bed is calming and soothing. Other teas to consider are lime flower, which is especially beneficial for young children, and lavender, which is particularly suitable where there is gut tension or spasm. Of course, all the previously mentioned herbal tinctures may also be taken as a tea. No one can deny the benefits of actually preparing a 'proper cup of tea'. Boiling the water, preparing the teapot, measuring the herbs, pouring the tea into your favourite teacup, this is a rather therapeutic ceremony in its own right – quite Zen.

Herb pillows

Laying one's head upon a soft, silky pillow of lavender flowers or hops induces sleep and relaxation via our sense of smell (olfactory nerves) giving a profound sense of tranquillity. Indeed, the German-born botanist Baron Ferdinand von Mueller recommended hop pillows to 'overcome want of sleep'.

Bach flower remedies:
* White Chestnut – calms the incessant mental chatter
* Mimulus – minimises fear
* Aspen – reduces anxiety
* Vervain – encourages relaxation
* Walnut – breaks the insomnia cycle
* Mustard – dispels depression.

See CHAPTER FOURTEEN for a detailed guide to the Bach flower remedies.

Foods rich in tryptophan

Tryptophan is an amino acid and the precursor to the neurotransmitter serotonin, which influences mood and sleep. Rich food sources include: bananas, figs, dates, yoghurt, milk, tuna, almonds, brazil nuts and cashews. A pre-bedtime snack of a small bowl of yoghurt and banana, followed by a strong cup of chamomile tea, works wonders in calming a busy mind and promoting a good night's sleep.

4 | Relaxation techniques

Progressive relaxation

This technique involves the conscious relaxation of each muscle, starting at the feet and gradually working your way up the body. There are a number of very good relaxation tapes available.

Meditation

Just ten minutes a day is sufficient. Find a convenient location and comfortable position, and instruct your mind and body to let go. Give yourself permission to relax.

Essential oils

Use either in a burner or add a few drops to your pillow. Lavender, cedarwood, ylang ylang, sandalwood, rose and frankincense all have relaxing and calming effects.

Calming herbal waters

A microcosmic health spa exists in our very own bathrooms, and it is free with no travel involved! A herbal bath has just three requirements: a bath tub, warm water and the herbs of choice (see following suggestions). A great number of medicinal qualities from plants are absorbed through the skin when added to baths; they enhance blood supply to the tissue layer closest to the skin and, of course, there is the undeniably psychologically soothing impact of immersing oneself in a warm, aromatic bath, with scented candles placed strategically around the tub. Whole plant extracts, good-quality pure plant oils and (this herbalist's favourite method) chopped-up herb can be used. Simply pop the chopped herb into a small muslin bag, or in the cut-off leg of a pair of stockings, and place it under the tap as you fill the bath.

A valerian bath

This bath has sedative and sleep-inducing properties, and is best used at night. Place an infusion of 100 g of valerian root or 250 ml of a valerian tincture into a full warm bath, and gently immerse yourself in the warm water. For greater results switch the light off and light a few scented candles and relax. A few drops of lavender oil can be added to the water if desired.

A lemon balm bath

Lemon balm also has sedative and relaxing properties and can be used instead of valerian, especially if there is restlessness and nervous tension. And it has a far more pleasant aroma than valerian! Add either an infusion of 100 g of the whole plant or one tablespoon of pure lemon balm oil into a full warm bath.

It is interesting to note that the aromatic scent of volatile oils such as lavender and lemon balm is not merely a pleasant sensation but it also has medicinal properties. The volatile oils stimulate the olfactory nerves, which in turn send messages to the brain, altering the brainwaves and producing a tranquillising effect.

CHAPTER THIRTEEN

EXERCISE AWAY FATIGUE

A vital body is the result of sound nutrition *and* regular physical exercise. We can't have one without the other. We are definitely not designed to be in the seated position all day long. Our legs are made for walking and standing, not sitting; and our arms are designed for movement, not the fairly stationary position of keyboard tapping or fork lifting.

Exercise improves the tone and quality of muscle tissue and stimulates the process of digestion, absorption, metabolism and elimination. High-intensity exercise is as effective as drugs in treating depression, without any negative side effects. It increases levels of the neuro-transmitters dopamine, noradrenalin and serotonin, all of which have a positive effect on mood and energy. Exercise also strengthens blood vessels, lungs and heart, which means improved transfer of oxygen to the cells and increased circulation of the blood and lymph systems. If the brain is deprived of oxygen, the mitochondria in the nerve cells cannot produce energy efficiently. Likewise, the nutrients in your foods are only as good as the blood supply that transports them to your tissues.

This is where we reverse the rules! Act, don't think, that will prevent any second thoughts, any snooze button hitting, any little voices sabotaging your best intentions – 'I'm too tired' or 'It's too cold' – you know the story. Never contemplate *not* exercising and I guarantee that after six weeks without any self-defeating talk, you will be on your way to a permanent exercise regime.

The importance of not procrastinating was reinforced for me recently when I passed a sign in the window of the Vocational Language Learning Centre. It proclaimed, 'Excuses are the nails used to build a house of failure'. Procrastination is indeed a self-defeating habit, achieving nothing but anxiety and worry; it is far better to tackle the challenge head on. Failure to attend to health concerns today just means more days of unnecessarily feeling below par. So, let's be decisive and make an enthusiastic commitment to achieving our treasured exercise goals.

The best time to exercise is in the morning. It begins your day on an energetic note that will improve your energy reserves for the rest of the day – besides, it is good time management. Ask anyone who exercises in the morning how they feel after a work-out and I am sure you won't hear them saying, 'Oh, I feel awful.' Instead you will hear a resounding, 'I feel fantastic! I have so much more energy throughout the day.'

Another very sound reason for exercising in the early hours is there are very few legitimate excuses not to. The only other thing you may be doing is sleeping. And a sleep sacrifice of 45 minutes is a great trade-off!

The only way any exercise regime will work, however, is if you enjoy it. I can assure you that if I had to get out of bed first thing in the morning to leap over a set of hurdles (that word sends shivers down my spine after a rather misfortunate belly flop over a hurdle at twelve years of age), or compete in a game of hockey (the sound of two hockey sticks clacking together still raises the hairs on the back of my neck), my compliance would not be good. However, I can easily jump out of bed for an early morning aerobics class, a gentle run or a brisk walk. So, choose something that genuinely appeals to you and make a commitment to it. Forty-five to 60 minutes, five days a week is all that is required to substantially boost our energy levels.

If morning exercise seriously does not suit, find a time of day that does work; for instance, commit to a lunchtime walk or slot into the evening a 45 minute exercise spot that is non-negotiable. Put the tracksuit on as soon as you arrive home from work and GO! No thinking remember, just move. Don't let your will be lulled to sleep by habit, paralysed by inertia or swayed by distractions, doubts or fears. Begin at once any action you would prefer to postpone. Create a positive precedent.

ENTICING, EXCITING, EXHILARATING EXERCISE

Here are a few examples to stimulate your enthusiasm. What exercise would suit you? What would you really enjoy doing?

- Individual — brisk walking, running, skipping, swimming, cycling, gym work-out.
- Group — boot camp, running or cycling groups, aerobics.
- Competitive — touch football, basketball, squash, tennis.
- Dance — tap, jazz ballet, Latin dance, belly dancing, samba classes.
- Video — aerobics, Iyengar yoga, Pilates.

CONTEMPLATIVE EXERCISE

A fantastic activity that combines exercise and meditation is to choose a letter of the alphabet and, while you are exercising, think of as many positive words as possible associated with your letter. One of my favourite letters is E, so to kick-start the exercise (if you will excuse the pun): E is for exercise, energy, exuberance, exhilaration, enlightenment, enchantment, etc. (Yes, even et cetera!) I guarantee by the end of your 45-minute routine, your cells will be positively bouncing with electrified energy. Our thoughts permeate our cells. As Marcus Aurelius observed, 'the soul becomes dyed with the colour of its thoughts'. Focus on the same letter of the alphabet for a week, changing your letter at the beginning of each new exercise week.

Another inspiring mind exercise you can do while taking your morning walk or run is to focus on a particular colour. Choose a colour and as you walk or jog, purposely look for everything in nature that includes your colour: flowers, birds, trees. It is truly delightful to notice exactly how much colour there is around us – too beautiful to miss.

Try to look and really see and hear the beauty that surrounds us. It is not surprising to learn that colour and sound stimulate brain euphoria, which in turn, produces endorphins. Science has demonstrated that there is a positive response in humans, animals and plants to musical soundwaves and colours. Let's not only improve our health with lifestyle and dietary changes but also use beauty – in colour, music and gentle thoughts – to enhance our wellbeing.

CHAPTER FOURTEEN

BACH FLOWERS

Dr Edward Bach, the Harley Street physician and bacteriologist, developed a range of thirty-eight homeopathic remedies in the 1930s, prepared from extracts of flowers and trees, to improve health by addressing the negative emotional states of mind we so often suffer from.

There are seven broad emotional states that the Bach flowers address: apprehension; indecision; loneliness; insufficient interest in circumstances; over-sensitivity; despondency and despair; and overconcern for others.

These gentle homeopathic remedies represent a more holistic approach to disease by treating the underlying emotional and mental needs. Our state of mental health can have a major bearing on the cause, development and cure of many physical illnesses. If you accept the premise that we become our thoughts, or the idea that emotional stress has an impact on health, then the Bach flowers play a vital role in the treatment of fatigue.

Bach flowers are ideal for self-treatment, they are gentle and subtle in their effect, benign in action and can be used by anyone. The dose is four drops on the tongue four times per day.

I'll mention the ones I use extensively in the clinic to treat fatigue, but, of course, there are many remedies to choose from which may also be appropriate (see APPENDIX TWELVE Guide to Bach flower remedies, for a complete list of all thirty-eight remedies).

OLIVE ॐ When you're completely and utterly exhausted, physically and mentally; feeling drained, lacking zest and with no reserve strength.

OAK ॐ When you're on the verge of adrenal exhaustion due to constant pressure and overwork. The typical oak personality struggles on, despite illness or exhaustion, hiding their tiredness and despondency.

ELM ॐ If you're feeling temporarily overwhelmed by responsibilities. Although normally very capable, the elm personality is a multi-tasker who may reach a point where the pressures become unbearable, and feelings of inadequacy and despair begin to seep in.

SWEET CHESTNUT ॐ When there is a feeling of perpetual mental anguish. This remedy is for those who have reached the limits of their endurance and are on the verge of nervous collapse.

HORNBEAM ✌ For that typical 'Monday morning' feeling; when the everyday routine has become too much. This remedy is excellent for procrastination arising from fatigue and feelings of being overwhelmed.

WALNUT ✌ Superb for helping to adjust to transition or change; e.g. menopause/divorce/relocation, for breaking links with the past. Walnut guards against powerful influences, and is especially valuable for those a little oversensitive to atmosphere or easily disturbed by domineering individuals.

MIMULUS ✌ Fearful of known things, such as illness, public speaking or deadlines, particularly when overly tired and on edge. The mimulus personality is often shy and timid.

VERVAIN ✌ Treats extremes of nervous energy and an inability to relax – the perfect twenty-first century tonic! The remedy for the highly strung perfectionist who tackles too many things at the same time and whose mind is always one step ahead of the task at hand. Insomnia is frequently a result.

WHITE CHESTNUT ✌ Helps to banish or at least settle that persistent (exhausting) mental chatter. Ideal to use if finding meditation difficult. For those times when we become preoccupied with a worry or an event, and go around and around in pointless mental circles.

The Bach remedies can also be used by babies, children and animals. Vervain, for example, is the perfect remedy for a young child who will not settle at night, and aspen or mimulus are effective in treating the terrors of nightmares. Dogs with separation anxiety respond beautifully to a blend of mimulus, rock rose and walnut. Hornbeam and wild rose will help students experiencing hormone-generated lethargy and lack of motivation, such as difficulty in getting out of bed and any apathetic tendencies.

BACH FATIGUE BLEND

A typical example of a fatigue blend of Bach flowers would include:

olive
elm
mimulus
vervain

Four drops on the tongue four times per day. This remedy addresses bone-weariness, feelings of despondency, being overwhelmed and anxious – utterly exhausted.

Other Bach flowers could be added to this basic formula to address other fatigue-related issues, such as larch for confidence, hornbeam for lack of motivation, oak for relentless effort despite tiredness, and wild rose for apathy and lack of vitality.

CHAPTER FIFTEEN

SUMMARY — HOW TO OVERCOME FATIGUE PERMANENTLY

1 | The vitality diet

To optimise the nutritional benefits from your diet and increase your energy levels:

- always eat a high-fibre and nutrient-dense breakfast
- include alkaline-forming foods; increase your fruit and vegetable intake (preferably organic with a substantial percentage raw)
- decrease dairy and animal protein and limit fatty foods
- increase non-animal protein and high-fibre, complex carbohydrates
- vary your grains – do not over-rely on wheat
- use oils rich in EFAs; e.g. linseed, safflower, sunflower, and choose oily fish
- drink at least 1–2 litres of water each day
- decrease intake of stimulants; e.g. caffeine, alcohol, sugar

- check for food intolerances and other digestive disorders
- chew thoroughly
- slow down eating.

2 | Key nutrients in energy production

The following supplements can be taken to increase cellular energy production:

- multi-vitamin and/or B vitamin complex with at least 50 mg of each of the B vitamins (except folic acid and B12 which should be a minimum of 400 mcg and 100 mcg respectively); plus, if required, extra B5 and B6 for adrenal gland support
- vitamin C, 2–4 g per day in small divided doses
- coenzyme Q10, 30 mg three times per day
- magnesium 500 mg per day, ideally magnesium orotate 300 mg and magnesium aspartate 200 mg
- potassium 600 mg daily
- check iron levels and supplement if required, 15 mg iron diglycinate or ferrous fumerate three times per day, and re-check iron levels within three weeks.

Note: If you take significant amounts of any single nutrient or herb over an extended period of time, it would be best to have a comprehensive naturopathic health assessment so that the dose is individually tailored, and to take into account any interaction when combining particular supplements or herbs and pharmaceutical drugs.

3 | Nutrients to improve mental alertness
To enhance mental performance and memory, select from the following as required:
- choline 500 mg twice per day
- glutamine 1000 mg twice per day on an empty stomach, and/or
- aspartic acid 1000 mg twice per day, and/or
- phenylalanine 500 mg on an empty stomach once per day if depression is a contributing factor.

4 | Herbal remedies
To soothe the nervous system and support the adrenal glands, the following options could be considered (best prescribed by a qualified naturopath or herbalist):
- nervine relaxants and tonics e.g. skullcap, oats, vervain, hops, passionflower
- adaptogenic herbs; e.g. Siberian ginseng, withania, gota kola, licorice root.

To improve memory and concentration include:
- ginkgo, bacopa or rosemary.

If there is depression consider:
- St John's wort (see page 130 for precautions

regarding St John's wort and some pharmaceutical drugs).

5 | Exercise and relaxation regime

To manage stress, achieve good-quality sleep and feel rejuvenated:

- make a commitment to an aerobic exercise of your choice: 45–60 minutes per day, five days per week
- find a meditation technique that works for you: just ten minutes per day will do
- treat yourself to a massage: relaxation, shiatsu and aromatherapy options
- take appropriate nutrients, relaxing herbs and Bach flower essences to encourage restorative sleep
- time out – feet on the grass
- slow down thinking.

6 | Bach flower remedies

To address the mental and emotional aspect of fatigue consider the following:

- olive, oak, elm, hornbeam, vervain
- 4 drops on the tongue four times per day.

(See CHAPTER FOURTEEN and APPENDIX TWELVE for other possibilities.)

A lifestyle brimming with vitality, energy and radiance is within the reach of everyone. *Don't hesitate, you can do it.* It just requires focus and enthusiasm and, most importantly, a heartfelt desire to achieve perfect health.

Recommended writing

Food diary
Keep a food diary to ensure you are on track and have not, for example, had a temporary white carbohydrate binge (bread, pasta, cakes) that has accidentally become permanent! Four times a year and preferably at the beginning of each season, record each meal and all snacks for a week. Ask yourself is this a balanced diet? Where can improvements be made?

Personalise the anti-fatigue regime
Photocopy the summary in CHAPTER FIFTEEN, highlight the key areas that relate to you, and add your own requirements. Place it on the fridge door or in your diary to remind yourself of your daily routine and supplementation regime.

Personal priority review
Set monthly goals in terms of diet, exercise, work, relationships with family and friends, spiritual attention etc., and review what you have achieved at the end of each month.

A note of thanks and gratitude

Make a mental note or a private diary entry of all that is right in your life. What are you truly grateful for? What arouses a sense of great appreciation? Focus on all the positives.

Total health is a fluid condition – there is always room for improvement and refinement. What a truly wonderful challenge!

Recommended reading

Balch, J., *The Super Anti-oxidants*, M. Evans and Company, Inc., New York, 1998.

Brand Miller, J., *The G.I. Factor*, Hodder Headline, Sydney, 1998.

Chancellor, P., *Bach Flower Remedies*, C.W. Daniel Company Ltd, Essex, 1971.

Chopra, D., *Perfect Health*, Bantam Books, London, 1990.

Colbin, A., *Food and Healing*, Random House, New York, 1986.

D'Adamo, P., *The Eat Right Diet*, Century Books, London, 1998.

Dunne, L., *Nutrition Almanac*, McGraw-Hill, New York, 2002.

Haas, E., *Staying Healthy with Nutrition*, Celestial Arts Publishing, California, 1992.

Hoffman, D., *The New Holistic Herbal*, Element Books, Dorset, 1992.

Mills, S., *The Essential Book of Herbal Medicine*, Penguin Books, London, 1991.

Mindell, E., *The Vitamin Bible*, Arlington Books, London, 1984.

Murray, M., *The Complete Book of Juicing*, Prima Publishing, California, 1992.

Murray, M. & Pizzorno, J., *Encyclopaedia of Natural Medicine*, Macdonald & Co., London, 1990.

Reid, D., *The Tao of Health, Sex and Longevity*, Simon & Schuster, London, 1994.

Treat yourself to an inspiring new cookbook from time to time (local libraries are a good source) – look for vegetarian, macrobiotic or allergy-free recipes. It is entirely possible to cook a delicious cake or loaf of bread without dairy, wheat, sugar and even gluten. It's true! One of my favourite cake recipes is made with buckwheat and rice flour, sweetened with raisins and dates and blended with rice milk. (Great for large groups of naturopaths getting together!)

GLYCAEMIC INDEX

The glycaemic index is an indicator of the effect carbohydrates have, after ingestion, on sugar levels in the blood. Carbohydrates that are rapidly turned into glucose or sugar have a high glycaemic index (over 70) and cause a rapid rise in blood glucose. Carbohydrates that breakdown slowly during digestion have a low glycaemic index (below 55) and release sugars into the bloodstream at a gradual pace. Less insulin production means the pancreas is not overworked.

Glycaemic index 85–110%

Grain-based foods
Puffed rice, corn flakes, instant rice, instant potato, white bread, popcorn

Simple sugars
Maltose, glucose, honey

Miscellaneous
Beer

Glycaemic index standard = 100%

White bread

Glycaemic index 55–85%

Grain-based foods
Noodles, oat bran, white rice, brown rice, muesli, shredded wheat, semolina

Vegetables
Carrots, parsnips, corn on the cob, potatoes, turnips, pumpkin, broad beans

Fruits
Bananas, raisins, apricots, papaya, melons, mangoes

Glycaemic index 45–55%

Grain-based foods
Spaghetti (white), spaghetti (whole wheat), pasta (other), pumpernickel bread, all-bran cereal, wholemeal bread

Fruits
Oranges, orange juice, kiwifruit

Vegetables
Peas, pinto beans, sweet potato, baked beans, navy beans

Simple sugars
Lactose, sucrose

Glycaemic index 35–45%

Grain-based foods
Barley, quinoa,
oatmeal (slow cooking),
whole-grain rye bread,
bran bread

Fruits
Apples, apple juice,
pears, figs (fresh),
plums

Vegetables
Kidney beans,
Lentils, black-eyed peas,
chickpeas, lima beans,
tomatoes

Dairy products
Ice-cream*,
milk, yoghurt

Glycaemic index 30% or less

Fruits
Cherries, grapefruit

Simple sugars
Fructose

Vegetables
Soy beans*, red peppers,
eggplant, broccoli,
cabbage, lettuce, onions,
split peas, french beans,
haricot beans

Nuts
Peanuts*, walnuts

* High fat content will retard
the rate of absorption into
the body.

ACID/ALKALINE CHART

	ALKALINE FOODS			ACID FOODS	
FRUITS	Apples	Grapes	Peaches	All sugared, dried, sulphured, glazed fruits	
	Apricots	Guavas	Pears	Bananas, green	
	Avocados	Lemons	Persimmons	Cranberries	
	Bananas	Mangoes	Pineapple	Olives, pickled	
	Cherries	Nectarines	Pomegranates	Plums	
	Cumquats	Olives, sun-dried	Quince	Prunes	
	Dates	Oranges	Raisins		
	Figs	Papaya	Tangerines		
	Grapefruit	Passionfruit	Tomatoes		
VEGETABLES	Alfalfa	Cucumber	Parsnip	Beans, dried	
	Artichokes	Dandelion greens	Peppers	Lentils	
	Asparagus	Dill	Potatoes	Mushrooms	
	Bamboo shoots	Eggplant	Pumpkin		
	Beans: green,	Endive	Radish		
	lima, sprouts	Garlic	Sorrel		
	Broccoli	Jerusalem	Soy beans		
	Cabbage	artichoke	Spinach		
	Carrots	Kale	Squash		
	Cauliflower	Leek	Taro		
	Celery	Lettuce	Turnips		
	Chard	Okra	Water chestnut		
	Chicory	Onion	Watercress		
	Chives	Parsley			
GRAINS	Buckwheat			Amaranth	Oats
	Millet			Barley	Pasta
				Breads (except	Rice, white
				millet/buckwheat)	Rice, brown (lowest acid)
				Cakes	Rye
				Cereals (except	Spelt
				millet/buckwheat)	Tapioca
				Corn	Wheat
				Crispbreads	
DAIRY	Acidophilus		Whey	Butter	Ice-cream
	Buttermilk		Yoghurt	Cheese (all)	Milk, boiled, pasteurised,
	Milk, unpasteurised (cow, goat)			Cream	dried, canned
FLESH FOODS	None			All, e.g. chicken, fish, meat, shellfish	
NUTS	Almonds, unroasted			All, except raw almonds	
	Chestnuts				
	Coconut, fresh				
MISCELLANEOUS	Agar			Alcohol	Mayonnaise
	Honey			Chocolate	Preservatives, benzoate,
	Kelp			Cocoa	sulphur,
				Coffee	Soda water
				Condiments, curry, spices	Sugar
				Confectionery	Tobacco
				Drugs, e.g. aspirin	Vinegar
				Eggs	
				Jams	

FOODS PROVIDING 10 G FIBRE

Only foods of plant origin contain fibre – there is no fibre found in animal proteins, dairy products or eggs. Fibre intake should be 30–50 g daily.

Grains and cereals

2 cups cooked rolled oats
¾ cup whole cooked barley
½ cup bran cereal processed
5–6 wheat biscuits (e.g. Weet-bix)
3 slices rye bread
3 slices high-fibre bran bread
5 slices wholemeal bread
⅔ cup oat bran
1 cup barley bran
½ cup natural bran
3½ cups cooked brown rice
8 cups cooked white rice (easy to see why white rice can constipate)
5 cups white pasta (e.g. macaroni)

Vegetables

3 cups steamed mixed vegetables
2 cups cooked carrots
2 cups cooked cabbage
2 cups cooked broccoli
1 cup steamed spinach
2 cups cooked sweet potato
2–3 medium steamed potatoes with the skin
1 cup broad beans
2 large corn on the cob

Legumes

1 cup cooked mixed beans
1 cup cooked peas
1 cup baked beans
900 g tofu
1 cup cooked lentils
1 cup cooked chickpeas

Fruit

3½ medium apples
3 oranges
100 g dried figs
10 dried apricots
3½ bananas
2 passionfruit
400 g blueberries
4 kiwifruit
6 nectarines
2½ pears
6 prunes
200 g raspberries

Nuts and seeds

100 g almonds
1 cup peanuts
100 g pistachio nuts
¾ cup pecans
¾ cup sunflower seeds

Omega-3 content of seafood

High (more than 1 g/100 g)	Medium (more than 0.5 g/100 g)	Low (more than 0.1 g/100 g)
Atlantic salmon, mackerel, trevally, mullet, canned red salmon (brine/water), canned mackerel (brine/water), canned sardines (brine/water), smoked salmon	Trout, King George whiting, blue grenadier, bluefin tuna, golden perch	Shark, whiting, flathead, bream, flounder, garfish, gemfish, leatherjacket, ling, john dory, red mullet, scallops, oysters, snapper, canned tuna (in water)

No excuses really for not conscientiously increasing your seafood consumption given such a choice!

Mercury content in fish

Given the high mercury content of large fish, such as shark, tuna, swordfish and kingmackerel, it would be wise to limit the consumption of these fish to once a week. Pregnant women, nursing mothers and young children should avoid them altogether. The Environment Protection Authority has set the allowable intake of mercury at 0.1 ug of mercury per kilogram of bodyweight; this translates to one 198 g can of tuna per week for an adult.)

FISH FINGERS (LIKE YOU HAVE NEVER SEEN BEFORE!)

500 g boneless thick fish fillets (a vegetarian alternative follows)
½–¾ cup wholewheat, buckwheat, brown rice or soy flour
½–¾ cup soy milk
1½ cups lightly toasted sesame seeds, or roughly ground and toasted
* sunflower seeds*
chopped fresh coriander and dill

Cut fish into finger shapes, roll in flour and dip in soy milk. Repeat. Roll in seeds and herbs until well coated and bake in a moderate to hot oven for approximately 30 minutes.

TOFU FINGERS

Substitute firm tofu for fish and quickly sauté in a hot frying pan lightly coated in olive oil. Although the tofu fingers (or should we call them tofu toes?) will not have the same Omega-3 content, they are high in phyto-oestrogens, especially isoflavones, which are beneficial for cholesterol, hormone regulation and prostate health.

Some tips about seafood

Buy your seafood from a dependable source; preferably not a supermarket where it is sometimes dipped in a solution of nitrites and nitrates to hide any smell. Also watch out for fish lying on paper that is saturated with chemicals – many stores do this to preserve the colour.

Non-dairy calcium sources

How much calcium do we need? The recommended daily amount is 800 mg daily for adults. For those at risk of/with osteopaenia or osteoporosis; plus women who are pregnant, breastfeeding, or postmenopausal, this daily dose should increase to 1200 mg per day.

There is a wonderful variety of non-dairy foods that contain calcium in an easy to assimilate form; for example, green vegetables, nuts, sea vegetables, sesame seeds and tahini, salmon, sardines and dried fruit. It is reassuring to know that the mineral boron, found almost exclusively in plant foods, greatly assists the absorption and retention of calcium.

A sample of high-calcium, dairy-free foods

(For comparison, 100 g cow's milk has 118 mg calcium)

FOOD	Milligrams of calcium (per 100g)	FOOD	Milligrams of calcium (per 100g)
Parsley	255	Kelp	1093
Watercress	190	Wakame	1300
Dandelion greens	185	Kombu	800
Turnip greens, cooked	185		
		Tofu, set with calcium sulphate*	170–250
Spinach	140	Soy beans, dried	225
Broccoli, cooked	130		
Bok choy, cooked	125	Soy milk (depends on brand)	225
Okra, cooked	85		
		Sardines	200–250
Unhulled sesame seeds	1150	Salmon (canned)	150
Linseeds	275		
Almonds	254	Blackstrap molasses	650
Brazil nuts	180	Figs, dried	255
Sunflower seeds	100	Raisins	65

*A note on tofu: There is as much calcium in 125 g of firm tofu (or for that matter in ¾ cup of kale) as there is in one cup of cow's milk, but the amount of calcium in tofu depends on the coagulating agent used. Calcium sulphate and nigari (magnesium chloride) are the two most commonly used agents; tofu prepared with calcium sulphate will contain more calcium than tofu made with nigari.

Also try using the water in which (washed) eggs have been boiled to cook rice, pasta and vegetables. Foods prepared in this manner will have a moderately enhanced calcium content due to the residue of calcium from the egg shells.

Sample menu for a high-calcium, non-dairy day

This meal plan would provide approximately 1000 mg calcium. If the rice and vegetables were cooked in 'egg water' the calcium content would be increased.

Breakfast

Muesli or seed mix with soy milk

Lunch

Wholemeal sandwich with salmon or hummus, and salad greens (e.g. rocket, spinach)

Dinner

Tofu, bok choy and broccoli on brown rice; green salad; soy yoghurt and stewed rhubarb

Snacks

Dried figs, almonds, soy milk banana smoothie

STANDARD ELIMINATION DIET

Daily menu plan

(Choose from Option 1 or Option 2)

Excluded foods include dairy products, wheat, corn, baker's and brewer's yeast,
egg, peanuts, soy, chocolate, orange, tomato and refined sugar.

Pre-breakfast

Glass warm water with lemon juice

Breakfast

Option 1	Option 2
Oat and banana porridge with oat milk or rice milk	2 slices rye sourdough toast topped with ripe mashed banana and dates

Herbal tea

Mid-morning

Piece of fruit in season

Lunch

Option 1	Option 2
100% rye sourdough salad sandwich, add tahini or hummus for extra flavour	Large fresh vegetable salad with handful raw cashews or almonds; or small piece grilled chicken, olive oil/lemon dressing

Herbal tea

Afternoon Snack

Option 1	Option 2
Small handful almonds, cashews or sunflower seeds	4–5 dried figs or sun-dried apricots (sulphur-free)

Dinner

Option 1	Option 2
Grilled chicken or fish (use olive oil, and herbs for marinade if desired), julienne of steamed vegetables (include broccoli, carrots, beans, asparagus, zucchini) Dessert: Lightly stewed fruit (in own juices) or baked apple stuffed with prunes, dates or figs	Brown rice and lentils or chickpeas, baked vegies of choice (e.g. sweet potato, parsnip, celeriac, carrots, squash) with 1 tsp. cold-pressed flaxseed oil Dessert: Fresh fruit in season, e.g. bowl of mixed berries; custard apple and passionfruit

Water as required throughout the day. At least 8 glasses!

GLUTEN-FREE ELIMINATION DIET

Daily menu plan

(Choose from Option 1 or Option 2)

Excluded foods include all the gluten-containing grains: wheat plus rye, barley and oats, plus those foods excluded in the Standard elimination diet.

Pre-breakfast

Glass warm water with lemon juice

Breakfast

Option 1	Option 2
Buckwheat and banana porridge with rice milk *or* Buckwheat pancakes topped with banana	3 – 4 tbsp. seed mix (use rice bran as bran component), grated apple, moisten with apple/pear juice

Weak lemon tea or other herbal tea of choice

Mid-morning

Glass carrot, beetroot and cucumber juice; if too difficult plain carrot juice is fine

Lunch

Option 1	Option 2
Lentil or vegie burger and salad *or* Homemade vegetable soup with rice or millet	Baked potato in jacket with tahini or hummus topping, large salad – include plenty of rocket, endive, cucumber and beetroot plus small handful raw cashews or almonds, flaxseed oil/lemon juice dressing

Herbal tea (as per breakfast)

Afternoon Snack

Fresh berries (in season) or pear

Dinner

Option 1	Option 2
Kidney or adzuki beans with brown rice, steamed vegies with 2 tsp. cold-pressed flaxseed oil, tahini/lemon dressing Dessert: Baked apple stuffed with prunes	Grilled chicken or fish seasoned with fennel and lemon, stir-fried asparagus, zucchini, green beans and broccoli in cold-pressed olive oil Dessert: Fresh fruit in season, e.g. cherries, apricots, peaches

Water as required throughout the day. At least 8 glasses!

FOOD CHALLENGE DIARY

	FOOD CHALLENGED (1 type of food only)	SYMPTOMS (e.g. mood, abdominal pain, bowel, itchy skin, runny nose, sore join
BREAKFAST (single serving challenge food)		
LUNCH (1–2 servings challenge food)		
DINNER (2–3 servings challenge food)		

PULSE RATE BEFORE & AFTER CHALLENGE
(beats per min)

Before challenge .... *bpm*

5 minutes after .... *bpm*

10 minutes after .... *bpm*

Before challenge .... *bpm*

5 minutes after .... *bpm*

10 minutes after .... *bpm*

Before challenge .... *bpm*

5 minutes after .... *bpm*

10 minutes after .... *bpm*

CELLULAR ENERGY METABOLISM

The food we eat largely consists of carbohydrates, proteins and fats, all of which serve as fuel. To convert these food sources to energy we require certain vitamins and minerals that act as synergistic co-factors or enzymes. These vitamins and minerals are indispensable in metabolising food and sending the by-products such as amino acids, glucose and fatty acids to the Krebs Cycle, where ultimately all cellular energy is produced.

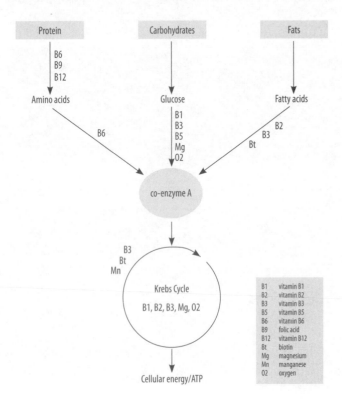

BRUSSELS SPROUTS ARE GOOD FOR US!

These delightful green bliss bombs are an explosion of vitamins and minerals. They are a good source of vitamins B1, B5 and B6, as well as folate, vitamin A, vitamin C, calcium, magnesium and potassium.

We have known for some time that the brassica family of vegetables (broccoli, spinach, cabbage, cauliflower and brussels sprouts) has a positive effect on liver detoxification, and its strong anti-oxidant characteristics have beneficial effects on cancer. Now we know exactly how it works. British scientists have discovered that chemicals released when vegetables such as cabbage or brussels sprouts are chopped, chewed, cooked and digested can prevent cancer cells from proliferating indefinitely.

Sinigrin, the chemical that gives the brassica vegetables their slightly bitter taste, is converted when eaten into allylisothiocynate (AITC). In an experiment conducted by the British Institute of Food Research, AITC was shown to interrupt the division of colon cancer cells. Instead of dividing indefinitely, the cancer cells float free and then commit cell suicide (apoptosis).

If you are not a brussels sprout fan, ask yourself why. I guarantee it will have something to do with an early childhood experience involving a soggy brussels sprout. Delete this memory and try again! Brussels sprouts are delicious. It's all in the preparation.

The shorter the cooking time and the less water used, the greater the positive effect. Two to three helpings of brassicas a week is recommended to obtain the health benefit.

Brussels sprouts, lemon and chestnuts

All amounts are approximate. Please vary according to your taste and hunger.

500 g brussels sprouts
10 – 15 chestnuts
rind of half a lemon
1 teaspoon whole fenugreek seeds
tamari to taste
chopped fresh favourite herbs; e.g. mint, coriander, tarragon

Lightly steam brussels sprouts and drain. Add a light coating of olive oil to a frying pan and heat, and lightly sauté the lemon rind and fenugreek seeds. Add brussels sprouts and sprinkle with tamari sauce. When slightly browned, add chopped herbs and continue cooking for a few minutes, then turn the heat off. Meanwhile place a small slit in base of chestnuts and boil for about twenty minutes. Remove from heat and run under cold water until cool enough to remove shell and inner skin. Chop roughly or keep whole (I like a mix of whole nuts and chunky pieces) and sprinkle over brussels sprouts.

This dish is heavenly served on a bed of fresh spinach with a dollop of yoghurt. Also gorgeous lightly dribbled with tahini.

TONGUE TALES

Tell-tale signs of a tongue analysis

SYMPTOM	DEFICIENCY/CAUSE
Quivering tongue, often short in length	Magnesium
Atrophy or hypertrophy of the tongue	Vitamin B12
Flat, sore, red and beefy	Iron
Glossitis (inflammation of the tongue), taste buds prominent on tip, sore	Vitamin B6
Inflamed, painful and sore	Folic acid, magnesium
Magenta tongue (purplish), flat, no bumps	Vitamin B12
Scarlet, raw, fissuring and sore – looks like car tyre tread	Niacin
Red, painful, cracked	B vitamins, especially B2, B3, B6 and folic acid
Cracks at corners of the mouth	Anaemia – iron and/or folic acid. Also could be a deficiency in stomach acid plus vitamins B2 or B6
Unnaturally smooth (often with ulcers), almost bald appearance	Folic acid or vitamin B12 or iron
Creamy patches (able to scrape off)	Oral thrush – infusion of clove as a mouth wash, acidophilus bacillus supplementation
Whitish patches (cannot be easily scraped away)	Leukoplakia or lichen planus – requires medical attention; folic acid, vitamin E, beta carotene, zinc and essential fatty acids
Brownish staining	Fungal – result of antibiotics or smoking
Enlarged vein under tongue and swollen gums/bleeding	Vitamin C (alcohol, drugs, cigarettes also factors); co-enzyme Q10 for gum disease
Feels dry either with or without a mustard coloured coating	Dehydration (test by pinching skin over breast bone, if stays puckered upon letting go indicates dehydration). Common in the elderly or where there has been a recent weight loss. Increase water plus potassium. May also indicate an iron deficiency
Dry with ulcers (no cracks); dry eyes and joint pains	Sicca syndrome (Sjögren's syndrome): an auto-immune disease of the connective tissue where salivary flow rate is reduced

THE POWER OF THE OAT!

The healing powers long associated with oats are derived from the grain's high nutritional value. Oats contain more essential fatty acids (EFAs) than most grains, and are an excellent source of B-group vitamins, iron, zinc, magnesium, potassium, manganese and calcium; as well as high levels of silica and vitamin E. Oats are rich in dietary fibre and high-quality protein. The outer coat of the grain, the bran, contains the B vitamin inositol in significant quantities. Inositol metabolises fats and cholesterol. Oats are quite high in the amino acids aspartate and glutamic acid, which we know have a positive impact on memory, mental alertness and stamina.

Oats contain vitamin K, essential in the formation of prothrombin, a blood-clotting agent. They are a good source of selenium, an anti-oxidant that helps to slow down ageing and hardening of tissues resulting from oxidation. Eating oats also helps your body regulate its iron stores as it contains the trace mineral molybdenum, which plays a vital role in iron utilisation.

As mentioned in our discussion of herbal medicine, oats are one of the best remedies for replenishing a depleted nervous system, especially in cases of nervous exhaustion associated with depression. They increase stamina and energy.

Oat home remedies

Oat tea
This tea is often prescribed as a remedy for reducing cigarette smoking, and other addictions. It also helps soothe inflamed mucous membranes of the stomach and intestines.

Oat paste
Oatmeal paste relieves the itching and swelling of insect bites or hives and

will also work as a poultice to draw out splinters. Indeed, an old-fashioned oatmeal bath can be used for any type of skin rash or itching.

Oat bath

To make an oat bath simply cook 1 cup of oats in 500–600 ml water for about 15 minutes. Place the mixture into a muslin bag (or a cut-off leg of a pair of pantyhose). Tie a string around the top and hang it under the tap as you fill the bath with warm water. Or use the bag of softened oats as a washcloth, squeezing the gruel out of the bag onto your skin.

Porridge

A homemade remedy to soothe your nervous system is at your fingertips: porridge! A bowl of oats is an excellent restorative breakfast that lowers cholesterol and stabilises blood-sugar levels. While porridge may not be considered a gourmet food, there are many ways of eating it that make it exceptionally delicious and appealing.

Some ideas to try:

- add a hint of almond essence
- add chopped dates, raisins or figs
- top with toasted sunflower or sesame seeds
- cook with apple, banana or pears
- dribble a spoon of rice malt or manuka honey on top.

Perfectly delicious porridge

2 cups rolled oats
4 cups water
½ cup raisins
⅓ cup each coarsely chopped almonds and sunflower seeds (dry
    roasted in heavy pan)
1 cup hot stewed apples
½ cup wheatgerm

Boil water in saucepan, add oats and raisins and simmer, stirring occasionally for about 10 minutes. Remove from heat. Stir in almonds, sunflower seeds and apple. Pour into bowls and sprinkle with wheatgerm. Serve with soy, rice or oat milk and/or yoghurt.

This porridge can be refrigerated and used as required.

Soaked muesli

½ cup rolled oats
⅓ cup water
¼ cup roughly chopped nuts and/or ground seeds
1 piece seasonal fruit

Soak oats overnight in water. Next day add nuts and seeds, and mix well. Chop fruit and add to muesli. Serve with rice, nut or soy milk. Add yoghurt if desired.

GUIDE TO BACH FLOWER REMEDIES

The Bach flowers are homeopathic remedies that address the major moods of the psyche, such as fear, despair, inflexibility and indifference. Choose remedies that match your emotional state. Up to five remedies may be used at a time. All the Bach flowers are perfectly safe. A few drops placed under the tongue or in a glass of water taken four times per day is all that is required. Subtle changes in one's attitude can be felt within a few days.

Uncertainty

Cerato
- unsure of self
- repeatedly seeks advice from others

Scleranthus
- indecision and hesitancy
- imbalance

Gentian
- depression from known cause
- pessimism and easily discouraged

Gorse
- depression of long duration
- utter despondency

Hornbeam
- inability to cope with daily tasks
- lack of strength

Wild Oat
- unsure of path in life
- lack of knowing what to do

Over-sensitivity

Agrimony
- mental worry and torture but appears cheerful

Centaury
- easily influenced and exploited by others

Walnut
- at times of great change
- sensitivity to outside influences
- link breaker

Holly
- jealousy and suspicion
- feelings of revenge

Fear

Rock Rose
- extreme fear and panic
- terror

Mimulus
- fear of known things, e.g. heights, poverty, poor health

Cherry Plum
- desperate and suicidal
- fears own actions

Aspen
- vague fears of unknown origin
- anxiety and apprehension

Red Chestnut
- excessive fear for others
- irrational anxieties

Overcare for others' welfare

Chicory
- self-indulgent and self-pity
- demands attention

Vine
- ruthless and inflexible
- desire to dominate others

Vervain
- extreme of mental energy, anxiety and tenseness
- inability to relax
- poor sleep

Beech
- ctitical and intolerant
- judgemental attitude

Rockwater
- self-denial and martyrdom
- high self expectations

Loneliness

Water Violet
- pride and aloofness
- desire to be alone

Impatiens
- impatience and irritability

Heather
- over concern with self but dislikes being alone

Insufficient interest in present circumstances

Clematis
- dreams of the future
- inattention

Honeysuckle
- absorbed in memories of the past

Wild Rose
- apathy and resignation

Olive
- complete physical and mental exhaustion

White Chestnut
- persistent worrying thoughts

Mustard
- deep gloom and depression from unknown cause

Chestnut Bud
- failure to learn from past experiences
- repeats the same mistakes

Despondency and despair

Larch
- feels inferior
- expectation of failure

Pine
- feeling of guilt and self-doubt

Elm
- overwhelmed by responsibilities and feelings of inadequacy

Sweet Chestnut
- mental anguish having reached limits of endurance

Star of Bethlehem
- for shock – physical, mental or emotional

Willow
- bitterness, resentment and blaming others for own mistakes

Oak
- effects of endurance when under pressure

Crab Apple
- the cleansing remedy
- self-condemnation
- over concentration on trivia

Rescue Remedy

For emergencies or accidents – a combination of five Bach flower remedies: Star of Bethlehem, Rock Rose, Impatiens, Clematis and Cherry Plum.

REFERENCES

Akhondzadeh, S., et al., 'Passionflower in the Treatment of Generalised Anxiety: A Pilot Double-blind Randomised Trial with Oxazepam', *Journal Clinical Pharmacy and Therapeutics*, vol. 26, no. 5, 2001, pp. 363–7.

Atkinson, R.F., *Your Health: Vitamins and Minerals*, Doubleday, Lane Cove, 1982, p. 147.

Bettelheim, F. & Marsh, J., *General, Organic and Biochemistry*, Brooks/Cole, New York, 1995, p. 607.

Bhattacharya, S.K. et al., 'Adaptogenic Activity of Withania Somnifera: an Experimental Study Using a Rat Model of Chronic Stress', *Metagenics Update,* August/September 2004.

Bhattacharya, S.K. et al., 'Anxiolytic Antidepressant Activity of Withania Somnifera Glycoithanolides: An Experimental Study', *Phytomedicine 2000*, vol. 7, no. 6, pp. 463–9.

Blackmores, *In Practice*, October 2002.

Bland, Jeffrey, 'Neurochemistry: A New Paradigm for Managing Brain Biochemical Disturbances', *Journal of Orthomolecular Medicine*, vol. 9, no. 3, 1994, p. 181.

Bone, Kerry, Seminar lecture notes: 'Phytotherapy for Chronic Fatigue Syndrome', 2004, p. 7.

Braun, Lesley, 'Recommended Dietary Intake . . . You are Not Getting What You Think!' *PhytoMedicine Focus*, 10th edition, 2004, p. 9.

Burgoyne, B., 'Adaptogens in the Twenty-first Century', *Modern Phytotherapist*, vol. 6, no. 1, 2000.

Canadian Centre for Occupational Health and Safety, 1997–2004 (www.ccohs.ca).

Edwards, C. et al., *Davidson's Principles and Practice of Medicine*, Churchill Livingstone, New York, 1995, p. 566.

Evans, Sue, *Notes on Materia Medica*, Instructional Design Solutions, East Lismore, 1996, p. 37.

Fischer, J.E. et al., 'Experience and Endocrine Stress Responses in Neonatal Nurses and Physicians', *Critical Care Medicine*, vol. 28, no. 9, September 2000, pp. 281–8.

Galland, Leo, 'Leaky Gut Syndromes: Breaking the Vicious Cycle', *Healthworld* Online, p. 75.

Gold, P.E., et al., 'The Lowdown on Gingko', *Scientific American,* April 2003, pp. 87–91.

Haas, E., *Staying Healthy with Nutrition*, Celestial Arts Publishing, California, pp. 48, 126, 279, 880.

Hunter, P., 'Herbal and Nutritional Support for Stress Management', *Bioceuticals Advanced Clinical Insights*, 2002, pp. 5–6.

Journal of the Australian Traditional-Medicine Society, 'Magnesium: A Review', vol. 17, issue 3, September 2001, p. 102.

Journal of Complementary Medicine, July/August 2002, p. 80.

Lyon, Michael, 'Identifying and Managing Food Allergies and Other Adverse Reactions to Food', *New Developments in Functional Toxicology and Gastrointestinal Rehabilitation, National Seminar Notes*, Series 2002, p. 50.

MediHerb Newsletter, April 1988.

Mills, S., *The Essential Book of Herbal Medicine*, Penguin, London, 1991, p. 518.

Mills, S. & Bone, K., *Principles and Practice of Phytotherapy Materia Medica*, Churchill Livingston, London, 2000, p. 534.

Modern Phytotherapist, 'Bacopa', vol. 5, no. 2, 1999, pp. 25, 31.

Nathan, Pradeep J., et al., 'Human Psychopharmacology Clinical Experiments', *Journal of Human Psychopharmacology*, vol. 17, 2002, pp. 45–9.

Nutrition Care Bulletin, vol. 12, issue 7, August 2004, p. 2.

O'Connor, Louise, 'Vitamin C: The Essential Nutrient', *Functional Medicine*, vol. 33, August/September 2004, p. 13.

Peverill, K.I., et al., 'Soils Analysis: An Interpretation Manual', *CSIRO*, Australia, 1999.

Reid, Daniel, *Guarding the Three Treasures*, Simon & Schuster, London, 1993, p. 46.

Roodenrys, S., et al., 'Chronic Effects of Brahmi (Bacopa monnieri) on Human Memory', *Neuropsychopharmacology*, vol. 27, no. 2, August 2002, pp. 279–81.

Rundek, T., Naini, A., Sacco, R., Coates, K. & Di Mauro, S., *Nutrition Care Bulletin*, August 2004, p. 3.

Seyle, Hans, *Stress in Health and Disease*, Butterworths, London, 1976.

Singh, Nalin, 'The Depression Debate' in *The Australian*, 12 June 2004, p. 19.

Soderholm, J.D. et al., 'Chronic Stress Induces Mast Cell-dependent Bacterial Adherence and Initiates Mucosal Inflammation in Rat Intestine', *Gastroenterology*, vol. 123, no. 4, October 2002, pp.1099–1108.

Turner, Vicki, 'The Importance of Iron for Preconception Health Care and Pregnancy, *PhytoMedicine News*, 9th edition, 2004.

Wagner, H. et al., 'Herbal and Nutritional Support for Stress Management', *Functional Medicine*, vol. 26, February 2003.

Weiss, Rudolf, *Herbal Medicine*, Beaconsfield Publishers, Stuttgart, 1994, p. 349.

INDEX